Cold Turkey Guide
To
Marriage, Family and Being Normal

Volume 2

John W. Ingalls

Many of these essays were previously published as a weekly column
entitled *Cold Turkey,* appearing over several years in *The Inter-County
Leader,* P.O. Box 490, Frederic, Wisconsin 54837.
Editor-Gary King, Manager-Doug Panek.
Essays previously published are used by permission.

Author photo by Drew Walsh. Used by permission;
Northwest Passage Ltd,
Webster Wisconsin 54893

ISBN-13:978-1981833566

ISBN-10:1981833560

Cold Turkey Books
27167 Engebretson Road
Webster, Wisconsin 54893
www.coldturkeyleftovers.wordpress.com

Dedicated to

Marriages Everywhere

May you learn to say
I'm Sorry with humility
and
I Forgive You with grace.

Foreword

My father once compared children to sheep. "Fence them in too small of a pen, and they have no room to explore or grow. Give them too much space, and they will roam too far from your safe and watchful eyes." A man of many sayings, proverbs, and words, his metaphor was most likely swept under the rug by me. Years later, having had a "sheep" of my own, there may be a shred of truth to it after all.

Now, my young lamb is only 16 months. An age where new words emerge weekly and every little thing is interesting to touch, and feel, and put in one's mouth. Some days I wish she really *was* a sheep, so I could pen her in to keep her from running off. I never knew a human who was only 2'7" with stubby legs could run so fast and disappear from your sight in the blink of an eye.

"Your life is about to change dramatically," many told my husband and I when I announced I was pregnant. And now, I look out into my living room and see how something so small impacts a life so greatly. A stuffed animal lying haphazardly on the couch, crusty with slobbery toddler kisses. Bibs, freshly washed, hanging on a chair to dry. Soft, pillowy hands and face to keep clean, safe, warm. A moldable mind and heart to teach and guide and pray to God that you don't screw up.

In many people's lives, there are a handful of moments that define who they are and who they become. One of those, I believe, is the moment you become a parent and suddenly you look at your own parents with fresh eyes. You weep from endless sleepless nights, you go through pain and confusion. Somehow joy brings tears too; you feel a tightness in your throat over something as simple as mussed up morning hair on a toddler, their cheeks flushed with sleep. And you think, "Did I do this to my parents? Did they feel the same way for me?" and most likely that answer is, yes. But just as importantly, you see your parents as human; people who need grace just as much as you do. You realize at many points in their parenting journey, they were just as clueless as you.

As I mentioned, my father is a man of many words. He would say just about anything to illicit a laugh from my sisters and I: a made-up song about a rich man buying a house and painting it "sorta blue", useless facts and information about trivial things, dad jokes to make your eyes roll all the way back into your head. There were wise words sprinkled in between the silliness, too. Words, like ink on paper, remain etched in one's memories forever. "Take it slow," he said to me, a nervous bride on her wedding day, an arm wedged into the crook of his reassuring arm, "this is the most important walk of your life."

And so, what happens to a shepherd once his sheep have become shepherds themselves? After years of his sayings and jokes being met with rolled eyes, scoffs, and groans from his four daughters, the old and wizened shepherd realizes his sheep have moved on to greener pastures. Therefore, a new flock must be created to entertain with tall tales and stories. Welcome to the flock, dear reader.

-Abigail Ingalls Roeller

Table of Contents

Introduction

Growing up is a painful process. So is growing old. We suffer through the bumps and bruises of early childhood and the humiliation of the early teen years. We seem to always want to be something other than ourselves. In the preschool years we can't wait to start school. When you are 12 you want to be 16. When you are 16 you want to be an adult. When you are old you want to be young again. When you are young you start to evaluate and measure your self-worth according to milestone accomplishments and years. It often begins with your grades in elementary school.

I was never really a great student but not a bad one either. I was in the half of the class that made the top half possible. My parents sent out Christmas cards outlining my progress. "Johnny says 4th grade gets easier every year."

Turning 16 was a big one. Coming of age and independence were defined by obtaining that all-important driver's license. If you couldn't drive, having a friend with a driver's license and a car was almost as good. The other way you tended to evaluate your progress through life was by your own physical development.

Junior High was especially harsh at revealing the differences in kids the same age. I had friends in my 8th grade class that looked like adults. I cringed in phy-ed class at my own inadequacies. Each night I would go home and stare in the mirror trying to find a chest hair. I looked so long that when I finally found one it was gray. I would use my dad's electric razor on the blonde fuzz growing on my upper lip. I hoped for a scratch or a small nick so I could explain that I cut myself shaving. I had two strikes against me. I had no chest hair and I rode the school bus until I graduated.

The years from 16-18 were special years. We knew everything and we were planning to do everything. We carried the impression, our parents knew next to nothing. We often compared notes with our peers to confirm our suspicions that our parents were really losing their minds. Even Mark Twain related his own experience. "When I was 16 my old man was dumbest person I had ever met, but by the time I had turned 18, I couldn't believe how much he had learned."

High School graduation meant higher education or entering the school of hard knocks. Entering this school was easy, graduating was tough. You just tried to make a passing grade and the teacher didn't grade on a curve. We learned that our parents really did know what they were talking about. Instead of telling them what to do and where to go, we started asking for advice. We didn't always take the advice but we were improving.

I have some concern that parents today (myself included) try to soften every blow and protect from every critical word, directed at our children. We don't want our children to suffer. We want them to have it all without having to work hard for it. It doesn't work that way.

Shakespeare may have stated that "All the world is a stage..." but I believe the all the world is really a classroom. We need to learn from and appreciate our own inadequacies and quirks. We need to realize that opportunity often comes in the form of adversity. We should view development of character as a milestone equal to the attainment of degrees, positions and bank accounts. Failure is as much a part of life as success. If we fall flat on our faces at least we are moving forward.

Most of life is defined by fits and starts. Marriage and parenting like career planning seldom follows a smooth path. There isn't an elevator to the top, we all need to take the stairs.

Volume 2 of Cold Turkey-Guide to Marriage, Family and Being Normal is just that-a collection of steps, stumbling up the stairs of life. Enjoy.

Birthday Presents

Gift giving is firmly engrained in our American culture. Birthdays and other special events prompt our generosity but the Christmas holiday has become a free-for-all. Shortly after our swimsuits are dry from the last swim on Labor Day weekend, we begin receiving Christmas catalogs. It seems our economy cannot survive without an all-out assault on our wallets at Christmas.

Gifts come in many forms and sometimes they aren't recognized as gifts. This past weekend, the weather was a gift. Despite the fact that we clearly need rain, the blue skies, and bright sunshine and brilliant fall colors were a true gift that couldn't be ignored. Not one to waste such a day I planned to spend most of my time with outdoor seasonal chores. We live on a lake so there are always waterfront duties to pick up and put away summer items. I went to my outbuilding and pulled on my chest waders. As my hand was reaching for the tool box somehow my fishing rod jumped in the way. I tactfully explained the predicament to my wife and she agreed to a diversion along the river just 5 minutes from our door. It was a wonderful gift of time together, wading and fishing and enjoying the fall colors. I allowed her the gift of catching all of the fish.

My children are also great gift givers. For my birthday, I was given a card and a cake imprinted with my age from last year. I guess that means I have another year that didn't count. In addition, I received a wonderful collection of photos with captions and comments about just being a Dad. The simplest gifts are often the most appreciated. Just sharing the lives of others is a fantastic gift that should never be taken for granted.

I don't mind receiving a gift; in fact, sometimes it is fun. I really enjoy giving gifts and I pride myself on giving the process some thought and carefully selecting the proper gift for the proper person. The truth is, for most people I delegate the shopping and gift giving to my wife who takes the job quite serious. She asks about the persons wants and needs and formulates a plan of action. Gifts are purchased, wrapped and delivered. It is usually after the gift is opened, someone will approach me with gratitude. "You shouldn't have..." they often pause and smile. "Thank you so much." I am usually left standing with a blank look on my face because I had no clue what they were talking about. "You're welcome" is my usual response and then I quietly whisper in my wife's ear, wondering who that person was and what did we give to them. She usually answers back, "That was your daughter and we just gave her a college education."

I can't easily delegate the gifting process for my wife to anyone else. I have tried over the years and I usually get caught. Sometimes I have conned my oldest daughter into assisting in the purchase of a birthday or holiday gift. She is a willing participant because she loves her mother and wishes the best for her. I have given up on buying clothes for her because they don't usually fit, or they are they wrong size, shape or style. If I must buy clothes I go for a one size fits all but that isn't usually appreciated either.

One year it came down to the day before my wife's birthday, Christmas Eve and I didn't have anything to give her. That's right, she was born on Christmas so if I forget to get her a Christmas present, I also forget to buy her a birthday present. Back then you couldn't just order it on the internet and expect express delivery. The internet didn't exist at that time. Being in northern rural Wisconsin, shopping options are limited, especially on short notice. Being a young husband at the time, I felt a strong need to give her a birthday gift and so with a modified sense of desperation I went to the local gas station that also had various items for sale. I chose carefully and wondered at her sense of delight on Christmas morning.

That morning she carefully unwrapped the chosen gift. Her smile faded into a sense of bewilderment. There in the box was a shiny new two-quart stainless steel thermos bottle.

"You shouldn't have..." She was right, I shouldn't have.

Bring Home the Bacon

The days when summer begins its slow descent from the hot, sultry nights into the cool mornings of early fall, I find myself in a happier mood. I love summer and all it has to offer but there is really something about fall that soothes my soul. I was born in September so that may be part of it. Apparently, I didn't want to show myself until the maples were red and the sky was a deep blue. I love the smell of crunchy brown leaves underfoot and the crispness of the autumn air.

The fall season kicks off with one of my best holidays. One of my all-time favorite holidays is Ground Hog's Day. It officially marks the second of February which we all know is a red-letter day. Equally important although less well known is International Bacon Day which occurs this year on September 3rd. Somehow Labor Day seems to get all the glory but International Bacon Day shouldn't be overlooked. It is somewhat like comparing Thanksgiving and Christmas. Christmas gets all of the glitter and glamor while Thanksgiving is often overlooked. We start hearing Christmas shopping advertisements shortly after International Bacon Day but we never hear about Thanksgiving until about the middle of November.

Actually, I am glad these holidays aren't celebrated with shallowness and lack of feeling. That allows us true believers to celebrate these designated days for what they really mean. Thanksgiving isn't "Turkey day" but rather "Thanksgiving" day. It is a day to give thanks and to be thankful for all that we have. It is hard for Madison Avenue to sell you a bunch of junk when the focus is on being thankful and spending time with friends and family. Likewise, International Bacon Day is about bacon and if you want to eat it with friends and family, that is up to you.

While you are preparing for International Bacon Day here are a few facts to help you get ready. The smell of bacon is alluring. Bacon cologne was originally invented in 1920, in Paris by a butcher named John Fargginay. He discovered what we all know to be true today; bacon scent is more powerful than anything Calvin Klein can make up. Any woman should know that rubbing a bit of maple-cured, smoked pork fat on the neck can call their man from afar. No longer do you need to labor over "honey-do" lists and nagging. Simply rub it on and wave a bit of crispy side pork before his eyes and he will be putty in your hands. If you want to keep the magic alive then feed him bacon and eggs for breakfast, a BLT loaded with extra bacon at lunch and of course a bacon, double cheese burger at supper. Don't forget to eat healthy, so a salad with bacon bits never hurts either.

Bacon has become so important to us that we often take it for granted. It has become part of our day to day lives and we tend to overlook its significance. Each year in the US we eat about 2 billion pounds of bacon, most of it at breakfast. BLT's became popular when fresh fruits and vegetables were more available to the public. Before that we just ate bacon sandwiches. There are about 25000 people in the United States with the last name of Bacon, who couldn't love a name like that.

Bacon is also part of an idiom that signifies success. We may call the workers of the world "bread winners" but in truth we are more delighted when they "bring home the bacon". How many of us remember those provocative television ads for Enjoli perfume, with the woman singing how she can "bring home the bacon, fry it up in a pan and never, never let you forget you're a man". I don't know if this perfume is still available but it might have been more effective it actually contained essence of bacon. On International Bacon Day, make sure you bring home a greeting card and some bacon because if you ask your spouse "what's shakin' bacon" but you don't bring home the bacon, you won't be makin' bacon and then nothing is going to save your bacon.

Bubble Wrap

Having grown up in the late 50's, 60's and 70's it should come as no surprise to anyone that there have been a few changes in the world around me. Obviously there have been tremendous technological changes in the past 50 years. Computers once relegated to research labs and NASA are now ubiquitous in our daily lives. The average American now watches television transmitted from a satellite, receives telephone and data transmissions via satellite and navigates an automobile under the guidance and direction of a GPS. However, some of the greatest advances have come in the areas of safety.

I am a strong advocate of safety and I strongly advise against risk especially when it involves my children or my grandchildren but at times I wonder if our efforts to protect runs a fine line with over protection. But as the saying goes, "It is better to be safe than sorry" to which I whole heartedly agree. Maybe it is my perception but sometimes I think we bubble wrap our kids just a bit too much.

I grew up in an age before seat belts, child car seats, bicycle helmets, air bags and smoke alarms. There is no doubt these have saved many lives and prevented needless suffering. But I also played with sharp objects. I had a knife that I carried in my pocket from the time I was 8 or 9. I chopped wood with an ax and not just for fun but also to heat our home. In the summer I left the house in the mornings barefoot and on a bicycle and often didn't come home until night. I went swimming immediately after eating and I laughed when drinking root beer until it came out my nose. By today's standards this was dangerous living.

Yet there is something wonderful about being a child especially the general lack of fear. When confronting a computer or electronic device for the first time, most adults hold back and tentatively tap at the keyboard, fearful of making a mistake or causing irreparable harm to the device. Not so with children. Most kids of any age plunge forward without fear quickly mastering anything put before them. It is often the same with other areas of experience as well.

Downhill skiing is another experience where children tend to throw caution to the wind and fly down the hills and mountains with reckless abandon. Parents, even those with experience soon find themselves slipping, sliding and snowplowing down the mountain behind their fearless offspring. Perhaps it is fear that holds us back but it is the lack of fear that sets them free. Now I am not advising unsupervised activities in dangerous situations which of course are foolhardy but I do think we could all learn something from our kids.

We recently returned from an adventure in Costa Rica and it was there that we met a young man whom I will call Mr. T. His first name started with T but I can't remember how to spell it so I will simply refer to him as Mr. T because it suits him well. Many of us can recall a television series a number of years ago that featured a brash character with an attitude wearing excessive gold jewelry named Mr. T. Our young man was better than him; in fact, he was a bit more like Crocodile Dundee in a pint-sized body. Perhaps about 5 or 6 years old, he was capable of taking on anything in his little world.

I never saw young Mr. T wear anything other than shorts, never a shirt or shoes. He was completely oblivious to the thorns and spiders and poison dart frogs in the natural environment surrounding his home. On a path near his home there was a sign that read "Snake crossing please use a flashlight" thankfully he couldn't read because he didn't have a flashlight.

While white water rafting near the home of Mr. T we crossed under a single cable stretched from one side of the river to the other. On one bank the cable was attached to a large pole. There was a ladder leaning against a wooden platform about 8 or 10 feet up from the ground. Attached to the cable by small wheels was a metal cage without any sides. We inquired about the use of such a device.

It seems this was the means by which a child and his or her friends would cross the river in order to go to school. A student perhaps the age of 7 or 8 or even 10 would climb into the cage and pull themselves across the river, hand over hand until they got to the other side and then send the cage back for their friends. This was not a lazy river. In the dry season it was fast and challenging, in the rainy season it could be furious and deadly. I can't imagine sending one of my children across the river on the "school bus". However, the government has decided to upgrade their transportation system and they did install a swinging suspension bridge now supported by not one cable but four above the same raging river. How is that for a bit of bubble wrap.

The Miracle Deer

The art of hunting deer has evolved from a relaxed outing into a highly technical endeavor. What was once a random stroll in the woods and fields has turned into a high-tech process resembling a Special Forces operation. Hunters now scout for deer with infrared cameras after carefully reviewing aerial photos to plan strategic ambush points. Food plots and mineral licks are developed to improve the quality of the deer being hunted and then the actual hunts are sometimes recorded for later viewing or sharing with others. Despite all of these technical investments and efforts, patience remains the key ingredient for success. When you add in the unknown factor of hunting with a child, patience becomes doubly important.

I enjoy hunting each fall, usually spending many hours afield during the whitetail archery hunting season here in Wisconsin. The season starts in sunny warm, September and extends into early January, allowing for plenty of unhurried time to relax and observe wildlife.

My youngest daughter, Billie Kay wanted to accompany me on a hunt. At the time she was in her early elementary years, so we planned carefully to have a safe and enjoyable outing. We picked a day with favorable temperatures because little hands and feet get cold easily. Secondly, we packed a lunch including hot chocolate, sandwiches and of course, snacks. Her extensive meal planning led one to believe, we were going on an extended family reunion picnic not a short afternoon deer hunt. Once the food was carefully tucked into our backpack, we added extra mittens, hats, scarves along with books and a packable doll.

Arriving at the woods, I slipped the bulging backpack onto my shoulders as if going on a safari while my perky third-grader smiled at me with big eyes and rosy cheeks. She held my hand and chattered constantly as we hiked down the trial to our deer stand.

"We need to be quiet now." I said in a low voice, hoping she would understand that quiet was supposed to last more than five minutes.

"OK, Dad. You're the best dad. Thanks for taking me hunting." I smiled back and nodded quietly.

"When we get there, can I have some hot chocolate?" She asked.

"Yes, of course. That's why we brought it along" I said.

Our arrival at the hunting spot was broadcast across most of the county but I resigned myself to just enjoy the time together. We carefully climbed the ladder into the deer stand and as we were trying to get settled into the place the backpack fell out of the stand crashing down the ladder and onto the frozen ground. In the quiet, snowy woods, the noise was no less startling than a car crash. I retrieved the backpack with our supplies and again attempted to get things arranged in the small deer blind.

After some careful maneuvering we were finally settled into place as I anticipated a few moments of peace and quiet. Two minutes passed in silence when I felt a small hand tapping my arm.

"Are we going to go down on the ground now and have a picnic?"

I smiled back, looking into big expectant eyes. "No, but we can have a picnic right up here in the tree, and you know what? If we see a deer today it will be a miracle."

"Wow! Really? I've never seen a miracle before!"

Somewhere between the hot chocolate, the cookies and the doll we looked up to see a deer approaching through the cold, snowy woods. She sat still without blinking and I could barely hear her whisper, "See Dad, it's a miracle."

I reflect back on that day and realize, the miracle wasn't seeing a deer, it was spending a very special time with my daughter. I was the one changed. I rediscovered how spending time with your child gives you a totally different perspective. We didn't bring home a trophy that day but the memories we shared are far more valuable.

Closet Archeology

Vacation travel today is significantly more complex than it was 20 or 30 years ago. For international travel item number one is a current passport but many other items are considered a necessity. I am currently in the midst of planning a Canadian fishing trip. Years ago, you crossed the border with a smile and a wish for fishing success. Now you are screened by homeland security, photographed, searched, x-rayed and finally interrogated by the grim reaper bearing loaded weapons on each side of the border.

If you are fishing in Ontario you not only need a fishing license but also an embossed natural resources card that costs about 50 bucks and expires in 3 years. It is sort of like buying a permit so you can buy a license. It was for this particular card I was searching when I discovered a forgotten portion of my past.

It is said of all of us that we have skeletons in our closets but I keep my skeletons at the office. I have a dresser drawer that is small and limited to junk. Most of what has accumulated in the back of the drawer are items that I don't know really know where to put. I have a few buffalo nickels each worth 20 or 30 cents and a couple of Morgan silver dollars. My passport is there along with my expired passport with a couple of holes punched through the pages. Old birthday cards and Father's Day cards from my children, some of them more than 20 years old were rediscovered, like old treasure unearthed from a sunken ship. I laughed how the children, now adults, scribbled with purple crayons and misspelled words that meant so much. "Congradulations Droctor John" one of them read, for my completion from medical school. Another was a list of rules to live by that I had presented to my children, now many years ago. It had been reprinted and returned on a previous Father's Day for my own benefit. After reviewing my own directions for fine living, I believe I am still following my own advice 20 years later and thankfully they are too.

Various coins and paper money from five or six different countries was scattered among some forgotten receipts along with a few pictures of me holding fish from past adventures. There was also a roll of 35mm film that had never been used. I wondered if it was still usable and if I could get it developed even if I did use it. Another item for the landfill.

My wife, like most women probably believes that I forget holidays and birthdays but I really don't and I discovered something to prove how thoughtful I am, or was. There on the bottom of the drawer, tucked in the back was a Christmas card to my wife, unsigned. It was clear that I thought about her and clearly intended to give her a card and a gift that year. By my recollection this must have been 6 or 7 years ago. Anyway, the card was still good so I tucked it back in place with the intention of being on top of things this Christmas season.

Behind the card was a small package discretely placed in the corner of the drawer where it wouldn't be discovered by anyone. Opening it carefully I found two silver earrings with inset opals also destined for my bride. I sat for a moment wondering when and where I had bought these. Using my past forgetfulness to my advantage I presented the belated gift to my wife and I gained three extra "good boy" points that day.

I never did find what I was looking for in drawer number #1 but we have an anniversary coming up soon so I am going to spend some time cleaning out drawer #2. I just might find another unused card and gift in the back.

Heavenly Music

I felt the pain shoot down my leg. The doctor side of me analyzed the pain and checked off the possibilities. The macho side of me gritted my teeth and the husband side of me wanted to whine to my wife asking for a back rub. It was excruciating like a great white shark grabbing my leg and shaking it. I knew it was time to see a real doctor.

The real doctor looked me over. He poked, prodded, gripped, twisted, squeezed and shook his head. "Yup, uh...ha, well, hmmm..." He shook his head and muttered to himself. He started to use big medical words and I knew I was in trouble. "I think your do-hicky is being squeezed where it comes out of the little hole in your thing-a-ma-jig. Maybe it is just some rust on your fenders but we'll see." I nodded. "You need some tests." I knew when he mentioned my thing-a-ma-jig, it was serious.

While the tests were being ordered I was ordered to go on the rack. The rack was originally a medieval torture device that has been revised, in modern times, as a treatment in physical therapy. I limped into therapy and humbly subjected my frail body to the therapist.

She poked, prodded, gripped, twisted, squeezed and shook her head. "Yup, uh...ha, well, hmmm..." She shook her head and muttered to herself. I bit tongue to keep from yelling. A bead of sweat formed on my forehead and I exhaled slowly. "You need a lot of work. Do these exercises and see me next week." I grunted and wheezed as I got off of the rack. Humbly accepting my assignment, I limped of the room.

I once attended a conference about chronic pain management. Pain is hard to define. According to the experts, pain is whatever the patient tells you it is. We try to refine the definition of pain by using other adjectives. It isn't just a pain, it is burning, stabbing, gripping, annoying, aching, throbbing, shooting, lancinating, sharp, dull, quick and constant. When all of these hit you, it is hard to sleep, move, sit, stand or keep quiet. I groaned trying to stop short of whining. I don't like whining. I longed to be pain free but I have also seen the consequences of someone who feels no pain. It is far worse. I knew in some twisted way, the ability to feel pain is a blessing in disguise.

I had read about experiences such as mine. One day it hit me. The pain shooting, stabbing, burning pain was with me as I went to lie down. Suddenly I found myself unable to move. I closed my eyes trying to block it all out when I suddenly found myself moving through a tunnel. It was a bright tunnel and a breeze seemed to blow over me. I felt a brief rush of anxiety but I forced myself to remain calm. A loud ratcheting noise surrounded me and came from all directions. I felt myself moving in the tunnel. Looking upward I could see someone moving in the distance but they were upside down. I could hear a voice talking to me but I didn't know how to respond. The banging noise continued around me and then I heard the music.

I don't know what I expected, perhaps angelic choirs or classic music harmoniously wafting in the breezes. I listened again to be sure. One song blended into another and I understood. The emotional pain in my head grew as the pain in my back eased. I couldn't be sure how long I was in the tunnel, it seemed that time stood still. A minute seemed like an hour and an hour was eternal. I blinked back my own tears as the last of seven Willie Nelson songs were over. "Blue Eyes Cryin' in the Rain". I wasn't in heaven; I was having an MRI.

Color Vision

"I've been thinking..." If you are a teacher and a student said "I've been thinking...", you would be pleased. If your child said it you might be suspicious. However, if your wife casually mentions it, you might want to check your wallet. Her sentences are often punctuated with dollar signs. Such is the way our winter began.

I don't fear her shopping antics, rather I am pleased by them. My shopping and buying exploits, I admit, are worse. Yet I perceive my purchases as being necessities and hers as being something less than that. I am sure her perception is the exact opposite.

"I've been thinking about remodeling the bathroom." Now I am not that old but growing up in rural Wisconsin is different than an urban area. Remodeling the bathroom meant moving the outhouse to a new hole. Having full knowledge that I no longer own a privy hidden behind any of the shrubbery, I realized this wasn't what she had in mind. I dutifully listened to her ideas and then we had a discussion. I won't say it was an argument but it was a full-fledged discussion, of which, I allowed her to gain the upper hand.

First there was a parade of contractors through the tiny space. I quickly realized that it wasn't just one bathroom, but the enthusiasm has spilled over into two other bathrooms. Each of the highly skilled craftsmen scanned, measured, pondered and made little dollar sign scratches on their worksheets and smiled. "Yep! We can do that!"

Our first assignment was to find ceramic tile to match what was already in place on the rest of the bathroom. I felt this was going to be simple. Twenty-some years ago we had basic colors. Our bathroom tiles in use were blue and white. Not so easy. White no longer exists. I quickly discovered that there are now 47 different colored tiles that look like white but really aren't white. Now they sport names such as "Frosty" or "Bleached Bone" or "Norwegian suntan in winter". Blue is even worse. The numerous and varied shades of blue range from "Glacier" to "Midnight Charade". The basic colors, blue or white, no longer impresses the tile purchasing public; it now needs to be dressed up in order to make its way into the modern bathroom. I think we settled on a couple of names that would make a good movie. Something like "The Moody Blues meets the Iceman".

People who regularly color their hair have been doing this for years. Light brown is obsolete. Now you color your hair "Sawdust Twinkle" or "Dirty Blonde Surprise". Anglers are no exception. I have in my tackle box numerous fishing lures with colors such as "green pumpkin", "root beer", "motor oil" and even "electric chicken".

Since she had been thinking, it got me thinking as well. Now a guy needs a tractor. In my lifestyle there is snow to push around, firewood to cut, fields that need mowing and if your wife won't let you operate heavy equipment in the back yard then a tractor is a good alternative. I decided to do my research before making just any purchase. Having just survived the initial tile color assault, I knew she would first ask about the color of the tractor that I contemplated adding to my collection in the pole barn behind the house. I found out the tractor marketing people haven't fallen for the new wave of color evolution. Tractors still come in red, orange, green, yellow and blue. Solid, single name colors give me a sense of stability and substance. It will be an interesting day when the nation's farmers, the original salt-of-the-earth people are feeding the world using designer colored tractors. In the future you may find tractors listed as "Dew Drop on a Peapod" or "Honeysuckle Afterglow" or possibly "Scarlet Sunrise". Then we will all be looking at the world through rose colored glasses.

Curfew

Guiding our children through the various stages of their lives is a never-ending series of adjustments. Just when you think you have a grasp on what to expect and how to respond, the situation changes. They seem to go from toddlers to teens in a matter of weeks. In fact, adolescent behavior is best described as a toddler on hormones. Instead of saying "NO" to all parental suggestions you are greeted with rolled eyes, a grunt and a moody curled up teenager on a corner of the couch with a cell phone.

Early childhood is the easiest, that age from 4-6 months. It is at that age you can park them on a blanket and have a reasonable expectation they will still be there in 5 minutes. Once they learn to propel themselves it is all downhill. The second most pleasant time during the formative years of a child is from around the age of 4 through 10 or 11 years. It is during that time when every child is still your friend. Despite our own deficiencies that may be glaringly obvious to the world, most children in that age range want to be just like Mom or Dad. Many children in the elementary age years still have heroes. That is why they want to be astronauts, firefighters, nurses and kindergarten teachers. These are the people we all looked up to at that formative time in our lives. The other great thing about that age was bedtime. When you told them to go to bed at a certain time you could still enforce it without being seen as the bully of the block.

It is during the teen years when naïve parents are finally faced with one of the most difficult negotiations of their lives. Negotiations between Teamster Union representatives and business executives were never as fraught with peril as the teenager-parent curfew debate. The mere mention of a curfew to a sixteen-year-old is enough to induce emotional seizures, or as my parents used to call it-conniptions. If you don't know the definition of a conniption fit, it is best described as the emotional outburst of a teenager when you firmly state, "I want you home by 10 PM."

For inexperienced parents, it is always best to start early so you have some room to negotiate. If you are serious about the 10 PM time limit you will likely be confronted with a full force conniption fit. When the weeping wailing and gnashing of teeth has subsided to a sulky sobbing you can then offer a compromise. This makes you out to be the good guy if you can do this with tact. You don't want to be viewed as someone who can be easily swayed or manipulated. Once a time has been agreed upon then you have the difficult task of trying to enforce it.

"Don't you trust me?" is the usual response from the innocent youth who is trying desperately to escape your watchful eye. My usual reply was "Of course I trust you, I just don't trust your friends." This can lead to other discussions so it is best to ignore the legalistic defense of their best friends forever. Instead focus on the curfew, the line in the sand, that time in the night when your teeth will grind, your palms will sweat and your heart will flutter with each tire screech on the highway.

Some parents are trusting or gullible and they simply go to bed without a care in the world. My wife is that way but not me. In the early days I would sit in a dark room listening to the ticking clock while cleaning the dirt from under my fingernails with a rusty knife. It became too stressful and it caused my hair to turn white at a young age. Then my wife read about an idea of setting an alarm clock and putting it in the hallway outside your bedroom door. The idea is for the compliant child to return home on time and turn off the alarm before Mom and Dad were aroused from their fitful slumber. This allowed me to at least flail around in my own bed rather than pacing the floor for hours. The idea actually worked most of the time. For the noncompliant child the alarms usually start going off as soon as they walk out the door for the evening. How you deal with a curfew violation is entirely up to you that is another issue completely.

This past weekend we attended someone's birthday party. She turned a spry 75 years. Along with other friends we laughed, played games and ate too much well into the evening hours. Sneaking back into our own home we were confronted by our own 22-year-old daughter, "Where were you, I was getting worried? Why didn't you call me?" I smiled to myself, the tables have turned.

My Preceding Hairline

The older I get the more I realize how much better I used to be. I am finding out how tough it is going through the aging process. It isn't that I am afraid of growing older but I look back with a sense of loss, loss of form, loss of function and loss of hair. One advantage of aging is that loss is offset by gain so everything balances out. My loss of form is replaced by a gain in weight. My loss of function is replaced by ingenuity in finding new ways to do my work. The thinning hair on the top of my head is offset by increased amounts of hair coming out of my nose and ears.

Someone once told me that at the age of fifty, gravity takes over. I really didn't want to accept that concept believing that it was really mind over matter. If you didn't mind it really didn't matter. However, no matter what you may believe, truth has a way of rearing its ugly head and forcing the issue. You can tint, tone, and tummy tuck, you can face lift and liposuction but you will have to face the facts. Father Time is organizing a direct assault on your body.

Somehow a slightly wider waist and stiff sore knees are relatively easy to accept. I can't run like I used to and I am less inclined to enjoy cold weather but what bothers me the most is my hair. I am most shocked about my hair when I look back at my high school and army pictures. I had long thick dark hair. I had a hairline that started at my forehead and I could go all day in the sun without a cap and not sunburn the top of my head. My wife would run her fingers through my thick dark hair and it didn't fall out. Unfortunately, everything changed

Somewhere in my late twenties I woke up one morning and noticed a gray hair. It stood out like a weed in a perfect garden. I plucked it with aggression. The next day there were two and the day after that there were four. If you want to understand the concept of exponential change, look at my old pictures. My hair didn't gradually turn gray it was more like a snowstorm hitting in the middle of August. I went to bed one summer's night and woke up with frost all over my head. I went from black to white. Now if I wear white shoes I look like a Q-tip.

I never considered coloring my hair although I know it is socially acceptable to do so. I prefer to let nature wreak havoc on me and I will just accept the consequences. If that is the worst thing that happens to me I will be very fortunate.

It isn't just the natural bleaching process that interests me but I also find the growth of hair a fascinating event. I have a theory that hair continues to grow inward even though it may appear to thin on top of your head. Hair is analogous to roots in a potted plant. It continues to grow until it finds a hole like the roots searching for the drain hole in the bottom of a clay pot. How else can you explain the hair coming out of your nose and ears? As a plant becomes root bound it loses some of its vitality and drops its leaves. In the same way when our head becomes root bound we start shedding some hair on the top of our heads.

Even though I have accepted my white hair I have a habit of letting it grow too long as if I am trying to regain my old form. Longer hair doesn't help because the hair on the top of my head is thinner and on the sides of my head it is thicker and more bristly. Now in the mornings after getting out of bed I have a direct resemblance to Bozo the clown. Rather than dwell on my receding hairline I now look back on the old pictures and remember what it was like to have thick dark hair. I liked my preceding hairline.

Chicken TV

I am not a great fan of television other than NFL football and watching the Wisconsin Badgers. I have enjoyed Downton Abby this past winter and sometimes when walking on a treadmill I watch Diners, Drive-ins and Dives although this doesn't promote healthy eating habits. Lately my viewing habits have been a bit more limited usually to one channel, Chicken TV.

More than 30 years ago, my wife and I were rather firmly entrenched in the Mother Earth News homesteading movement. We had chickens, pigs, ducks, cows, a solar powered outdoor shower and we ate our own home-grown carrots with the dirt still on them. My grandmother felt sorry for us and gave us our first television. It had a small screen, fuzzy reception and was black and white. Prior to that time, we had to rely on one channel for entertainment, chicken TV. However, around sunset the viewing became quite boring when they all went in to roost. A couple of the bantam chickens were wilder than a pheasant and always roosted about 20 feet up in a tree next to the house. We were never quite sure where they were until 4:30 in the morning when the chicken TV converted to an alarm clock.

Moving off of the farm I was able to be free of the morning chicken alarm until now. For about the past ten years my wife has been asking for chickens. I have always agreed with her and I would bring home a frozen chicken from the store. More recently she has been more vocal and clarified her desires. She wanted live chickens in the backyard. Finally, I agreed to make her eternal wishes come true. We had a small unused garden shed full of some junk and her reasoning was simple. This could be relocated behind our pole barn converted to a small chicken coop. Almost no cost at all and hardly any work involved (for her). Between the wire, lumber, time, chickens and feed we now have our costs down to $17 for a dozen eggs. We sell them for $2 a dozen. I can see how America's farmers are getting wealthy.

I was certainly not in the mood to raise chicks. If we were getting chickens, why not start with experienced chickens, something that already knew how to cluck and lay eggs. Rather than some flighty pullets we found some middle-aged chickens and they even gave us a rooster for free. Why not, I reasoned. If he bothers me this weekend there will be chicken stew on Tuesday. He must have been about 40 in chicken years because he sleeps late, he is hen pecked and has no tail feathers and only one eye. In the morning he throws his head back and yawns. He hops around in a circle and cocks his head to look you over. He doesn't crow until noon and then only to impress his lady friends. My kind of rooster. Our grandchildren have named him Popeye Henry so I guess that means we are stuck with him.

One day our granddaughters were visiting and despite the nice weather, which seems to be exceedingly rare this spring, they wanted to watch television. When we were unsuccessful at trying to redirect their wishes I finally conceded. "OK, let's go outside and watch TV". I finally had to explain it was "Chicken TV".

We brought kitchen scraps to the pen and also tossed cracked corn on the ground to watch them scratch and peck. We opened and closed the chicken door, tossed around some bedding straw and picked up the eggs. By the end of the afternoon they requested that I build a bench so they could sit and watch "Chicken TV".

On Mother's Day they were so excited to come to Grandma's house for dinner and a movie, the chicken movie. While dinner was being prepared they parked themselves on the chicken bench to watch the show. After dinner was completed they returned to the same location with some table scraps and were thoroughly entertained. As it neared the time to go, Ella B. turned to Grandma and asked, "Grandma, when we are gone, do you come out here all alone and watch the chicken movie?" I am happy to report, yes, she does.

I guess there is finally something wholesome for the kids to watch "Chicken TV".

Driving in the Fog

I sympathize with the newest generation entering the work force. Uncertain political and economic times is unsettling enough for those of us who have made a mark in the world but it is doubly so for those just graduating. The educational process is great at developing the intellectual mindset but I have always felt it lacks true credibility at preparing one for the actual process of working.

One of our delightful offspring is struggling with career decisions. She isn't afraid of work and she has a good work ethic but there remains a serious and persistent level of anxiety about her entry into the work force. Uncertainty plays a role in this but perhaps we have failed her as well. Many children see their parents as stable and settled as if they had it all together. I am sure some young people can't believe their own parents were once awkward teens harboring the same insecurities they now have. After all, haven't all parents always known exactly what they were going to do in life and everything turned out exactly as planned?

My advice is easy but incredibly difficult to follow. Go for a drive on a foggy day. I have often related to each of our children that life is actually a bit like driving in the fog. You start out with a general knowledge of where you want to go but you make a thousand adjustments in the process. Only able to see just so far it is easy to become anxious when thinking about the final destination but that also is what makes it so interesting. Those twists and turns in the road and the detours along the way lead us to so many unplanned and expected joys that we never would have encountered if we had lived out the boring path we had planned.

My own life is an example. Born during that prosperous post war time I am part of a generation known as the baby boomers. The oldest members of this generation are now retiring and the youngest members are just beginning to figure things out. You see we were a free-spirited group of people that changed politics and the work place. We grew up during tumultuous times of the Vietnam War, long hair, psychedelic colors and the Beatles. For many, life wasn't just driving in the fog, we lived in the fog.

My point being, having our lives planned out just never really occurred to most of us. I planned to get out of high school and become a Mountain Man like Jeremiah Johnson. While making plans to head to the mountains I ended up joining the U.S. Army as a way to get there. Colorado was my home for 3 years but I found that I missed the lakes and woods of northern Wisconsin. My wife's educational efforts then lead us to Northern MN where I worked as a restaurant assistant manager. At least that was my title but I actually spent most of my time chopping lettuce and grilling steaks for others.

Going to medical school wasn't even considered. Living my life in the fog I was destined to make many adjustments on my road in life. Never quite satisfied with my status quo I was forever searching. I was never certain about that for which I was searching but I kept looking anyway. Along the way I cleaned chimneys, cut brush on the roadways, cleaned milk trucks at Burnett Dairy, worked for Johnson Lumber delivering sheetrock and shingles, was a traveling bird feeder salesman, insulated chicken houses and attics, and did field work for a farmer. We even had our hand at homesteading where we raised our own vegetables, chickens, ducks, pigs and cattle.

Reflecting back, I am glad I never really had it all figured out. I am happy for all of the young people now considering their future positions in this world. It is comforting to know many of them have it all written down and cast in stone. I am surprised at the turns my life has taken. I went places and did things I would never have considered possible and not because I planned it out. One day I just started driving in the fog and found out that I really enjoyed the ride.

Face Plant

I failed in my quest to be the last member of my family to graduate from a dumb phone to a smart phone. I have been firmly entrenched in the flip phone era, the kind of phone that is simple and cheap and is generally durable. The kind of phone you use to actually talk to others. However, durability has its limits and now I must make a decision if I want to remain connected to the rest of my family. I really don't have a great problem remaining disconnected but in the interest of family unity the issue has been forced upon me.

I never intended to ruin my phone it just happened. Tammy had this great idea to get a paddle board. It is in the image of a surf board with a small rudder at the back. It is similar to a canoe without sides or seats and you stand and use an oversized paddle to propel yourself across the water. The profile of the board is so low that it gives the illusion of someone walking on water. I prefer to call it a water board which is reminiscent of an outlawed method of torture. Now on calm sunny days and quiet evenings she can be seen effortlessly skimming across the water on her new water board.

It was last evening when the sun was setting and the frogs were just beginning to sing that I decided to try it. I had managed to uneventfully cruise around in the shallows without serious mishap. My wife and daughter just completed an expedition length cruise along the shore and I decided to give it another try. Since I had successfully negotiated the craft on my previous attempts I decide to forego the bother of changing into appropriate swimming attire, I simply stepped barefoot onto the back of the board after tightening the Velcro tether around my ankle. I stood a bit too far back and the water lapped about my feet as the front rose up to meet the waves.

My spectators implored me to move forward on the board so it would be more stable. Walking on land and water are two different things. Moving forward on the board which is suspended between earth and sky is no simple task. As I stepped forward the board promptly exited to the rear. For a brief moment I hung over the water in suspended animation as a cartoon character waiting for the inevitable debacle. It came.

The cool water embraced me as I plunged face first into the lake. I made no attempt to right myself, it was hopeless. As I arose from the depths I was greeted with unbridled mirth and rapturous chortling from my audience. To bring such joy to ones' family is not without expense and that expense was a complete destruction of any self confidence in my water boarding ability. I stood in the water, wet clothes clinging to my less than stellar physique. It was then my daughter pointed out the wet plastered outline of my cell phone in my pocket.

To dry out a wet phone I was told to take it apart and bury it into a bag of rice. The idea is for the uncooked rice to absorb the water and restore your highly valuable technical device to its former glory. I was creating techno-sushi; chop suey with a ring tone. I set the phone on the table and the screen went black as the phone started convulsing. It went into a constant buzz and began moving around the table like a blind cockroach. I put it out of its misery. Someone told me to try and bake it in the oven at 250 degrees until it dried out. I didn't try. Once I had a watch that suffered from a moisture overload and I tried to dry it out in a frying pan. I melted it. I needed a cell phone you could dunk and bake, sort of like the old Timex watches that take a licking and keep on ticking.

The next morning at breakfast I decided to reward myself with a good breakfast before heading off to work. I made a platter of French toast smothered with butter and syrup as I queried the internet searching for another cell phone option. My wife, always the one to recognize discrepancies in my appearance pointed out that I had a spot of butter on my forearm. Using my finger, I wiped it off and licked my finger. It turned out to be shaving cream. Some days you are the dog and some days you are the hydrant.

Fashion Statements

It is very unlikely that I would ever be considered as an example of the latest fashions. I am firmly entrenched in my own little world and am not easily swayed by new ideas on how to dress. In fact, I am not impressed by the newest or latest fad. I lean somewhat toward traditionalist thinking but that doesn't mean I am completely against change. But I would rather accept change on my own terms.

As a bit of background, I grew up on the 60's and 70's which is so "last century" but interestingly some of those same fashion ideas are now starting to reemerge. Old is now new. Traditional names are equally or more popular than hyphenated designer names among our newborns today. Matilda could be your great-grandmother or your niece. Along with names, hair is also making a comeback. I tend to like longer hair probably because I am losing it in patches. Long hair for me now means it is sticking out of my nose or growing on the top of my ears and it needs to be plucked or trimmed. However, I could be equally comfortable with long or short hair, I have no problems with the resurgence of longer hair styles.

Tattoos and body piercings have been an area I am unwilling to embrace. Outside of military service, when I was in my formative years, multiple tattoos were associated with a fringe of society. Not so today. Tattoos have been widely accepted among our youth and mainstream adults. It isn't uncommon to see young professionals with skin art covering more of their skin than their clothing. I haven't been willing to jump into that line of fashion. If I ever do decide to get a tattoo it will read "Do Not Resuscitate" and will be in bold letters across my chest. I guess that wouldn't be a fashion statement so much as it represents my advance directives. Instead of a tattoo, a magic marker would work just as well.

Piercings creep me out just a bit. I can understand pierced ears and maybe even a nose stud but anything beyond that leaves me with more questions than answers. Lips and eyebrow piercing is a bit more troubling to me but when you get to nipples and genitals I start to have shivers down my back. The piercing that bothers me the most is the tongue stud. Perhaps I can understand some aboriginal warrior who pierced his tongue with the sharp bone of a wild beast because he was trying to appease the gods of the forest but when we can sit in a comfortable chair and have the wisdom of the ages at our finger tips why would anyone want to shove a sharp nail through the middle of their tongue? These same individuals would likely decline a vaccination because they don't like needles. Go figure.

Tongue studs and tattoos are all on my list of things to avoid but the one fashion statement that really makes me wonder is the baggy pants with the crotch somewhere above your ankles look. I am not judging the people who prefer to wear their clothing this way, I just fail to see any possible reason why I would choose that style over any other clothing option. I can get along in most social settings and I can adjust from a business suit to jeans and a camo T-shirt with equal ease but I could never see myself in the baggy pants look. I would rather live and work in long hair and wear a polyester leisure suit with a wide paisley tie and stripped bellbottom pants that wear size 58 trousers sagging around my knees. Call me traditional.

Fatherly Advice

In my experience it is not uncommon to have young people approach me for career advice. The seeker of advice may be well informed or may be entirely naïve about the subject of their inquiries but the fact that they are asking is a decidedly good thing. Getting and giving good advice is always welcome in my way of thinking, however receiving negative advice may prove to be the more valuable.

My wife and I have had the wonderful, albeit expensive task of assisting our 4 now grown daughters through career choices and University education. It wasn't always easy. Scholarships were limited, grants seemed to evaporate and offers for loans seemed a bit too easy as long as you put up your car, kid, house and a kidney as collateral. That left work as the only realistic option of success in the long run. My wife changed jobs to help pay for some of the college expenses. At her current salary if we applied all of her earned income before taxes just to college expenses for 4 girls attending a private college in the Midwest it would take her 21.33 years of labor. If she took out money for coffee and lunch she may never retire. Ah the joys of assisting the next generation.

The cost of education although serious isn't the main issue. Making wise and reasonable choices is the primary goal. You can gently offer advice or you can force the issue and each method may work depending on the circumstances. In our case neither worked as we had hoped. ACT scores seem to be an important consideration by some at the University admissions offices around the country. A higher score on your test often leads to a second look on the application. One of our children was convinced she wanted her scores sent off the far corners of the globe including southern California and the University of the US Virgin Islands in St Thomas USVI among others. I am sure these are fine destinations for advanced studies; they just didn't fit our way of thinking. She completed her application and carefully documented the given codes for each of her chosen locations of study. On the way to the Post Office box somehow the envelope was steamed open and the codes were changed to Midwestern schools most favored by her parents. It was nearly 10 years before we dared tell her of our intervention. Parental advice can be given indirectly and work just as well.

I was reminded again of fatherly advice at the recent funeral of my own father. Ironically, I remember little of the advice he offered because it was usually veiled in something called work. That is why I was stunned to hear of the story of a young man attending his funeral.

It seems he met my father at the golf course. Each would be considered social golfers, satisfied with a good stroke and undeterred by a ball in the rough or out of bounds. Thrown together by chance as each was golfing alone they struck a common chord. My father had completed his work years and left his mark. The younger was just the opposite, searching for direction with lofty goals and hopes but little foundation to support them. "Your father was so encouraging to me" he continued. "When I told him my ideas he simply told me to follow my dreams." He paused, "I wish I had the chance to have known him better."

I was dumfounded. I thought he must have talking about someone else he met on the golf course. My father may have been many things to many people but I never really considered him a career counselor. I reflected on what I had just heard. I remembered what advice he had given me nearly 40 years in the past. He may have told this young man to "follow his dreams" but he told me to "get a job and work hard".

It is hard to judge the value of advice when you first receive it but with the advantage of time you can look back and see it much more clearly. Following your dreams is wonderful advice but he gave me a foundation to shoot for the stars when I was ready to go and the determination and stamina to make it happen. Thanks Dad for the good advice.

Becoming Grandparents

Nothing prepared me for the role of being a grandfather. Mentally and emotionally I wasn't ready to accept the role. Physically I wasn't old enough, after all aren't grandpas and grandmas old and gray and slightly bent at the knees and back? I still had years before I could realistically consider retirement, I had a daughter in high school and I still had the mind of an 18-year-old. Then I looked in the mirror. What looked back at me was a shock. I now looked like every grandfather should look. I had gray hair for that distinguished look, a lightly expanded abdomen for that successful look and hemorrhoids for that concerned look. Maybe I was ready to be a grandpa. On the other hand, my loving wife was ready for the role of grandmother but she didn't look the part. Appearing 20 years younger than myself and sometimes mistaken for being my daughter she was ready to embrace her grandchildren with open arms.

Grandmothers are like mothers with a little seasoning. They have the unique ability to blend together love, forgiveness and a bit of discipline into a big bowl with some sugar and it always comes out looking like warm chocolate chip cookies and cold milk. Grandmothers and food almost always go hand in hand. Maybe that is why we eat when we experience stress because it subconsciously reminds us of the unconditional love that our grandmothers bestowed upon us. Even today certain food smells will trigger memories of my grandmothers cooking up huge pots of baked beans, pancakes or big turkeys for Thanksgiving or Christmas.

While grandmothers may be identified with a certain degree of reverence, grandfathers are often associated with character. Grandfathers sometimes have nick names such as "Gramps" or "Papa" but just as likely they may be known as "Crazy old Coot", "Geezer" or "Old Goat". These nick names often reflecting their own level of character development. Grandfathers also have two other traits that set them apart from grandmothers, the ability to tell stories over and over and over again and the second is the ability to stretch the honest truth beyond the breaking point.

Visits to Grandpa's and Grandma's house often follow a similar pattern. I see similarities from my childhood replayed in my children's experiences and now with my own grandchildren as they visit us. Grandma would meet you at the door with hugs and adoring comments about your new shoes or how your hair cut looked, quickly followed by comments such as, "My you kids look hungry, want something to eat?" It didn't matter what your parents said because Grandma was going to feed you anyway. You didn't dare to not eat because that might offend Grandma and maybe the next time she wouldn't make your favorite cake or cookies.

Grandma was almost always the first to greet you at the door, but Grandpa was more reserved or lazy. He would be waiting in his easy chair and would call out to you "Come here you little whipper-snapper", he would mess up your new haircut with his big hands and then pause. "Say, did I ever tell you about the time...?" You always knew what was coming because Grandpas can't remember if they told the story before and each time it was told the truth got stretched enough that it was never quite the same story anyway. When you are in preschool or grade school ages you listened politely and even beg for more stories. When you got a bit older you learned how to discreetly roll your eyes when listening to these stories. My Dad is a classic story teller and he has told enough tall tales that I noticed it was starting to affect my children. They rolled their eyes back so much that I thought they were coming loose. One of my kids can now move her eyes independent of each other like an iguana. I guess she can thank her Grandpa for that.

When I first became a Grandpa ,it frightened me. I wasn't old enough or wise enough to be a grandfather. I couldn't stretch the truth and repeat myself like a real grandpa could. And then one day it happened. My granddaughter Ella climbed up onto my lap, she gave me part of her cookie from grandma and said, "Grandpa, will you tell me a story?"

I cleared my throat, thought for a moment and then as natural as ever I began, "Did I ever tell you about the time..." I glanced down at her in time to see her smile at Grandma and then roll her eyes ever so slightly.

Feeling Wealthy

I pity the poor soul who has material wealth but no friends. It would however seem counterintuitive that those with cash in their pockets would be friendless. Yet money doesn't guarantee friends or loyalty. Friends or perhaps I should say true friends care little about your personal bank account and more about your true wealth. Those who have true friends are indeed wealthy.

We just experienced a fine dining experience combining friends and fondue. If you have never experienced a well-prepared fondue you are missing a treat. Fondue originated around the mountainous area of Europe that now comprises Switzerland, France and the Piedmont region of Italy. The earliest known recipe for fondue was recorded in Zurich dating back to 1699 which was a recipe for cheese melted with wine in which bread was dipped. Fondue in its simplest form is simply meat or other various types of food skewered on a stick or fork and placed into a communal pot of liquid. This may include but isn't limited to, cheeses, hot oil or chocolate. In our case it included all three.

The first course was spent in the kitchen, laughing, eating, drinking, talking and more eating. Vegetables and fruit coated with a delicious cheesy fondue set the stage for the evening. For more than an hour we spent time getting reacquainted with each other, inquiring about life in general. As the communal pot of cheesy dip began to wane we migrated into the dining room and feasted on fresh bread and a big garden salad with homemade green goddess dressing complete with a hint of anchovy paste. While the salad was passed our conversations continued and our hosts made sure we lacked for nothing.

Hot cauldrons of oil were centrally placed on our table and bowls of cubed beef tenderloin were within easy reach. Piercing one or two cubes of meat we placed our color-coded forks into the communal hot oil as we cooked our way through the evening. A fondue meal is perfectly suited for dining with friends. It is the antithesis of fast food. It is slow and may at times seem a bit tedious but it is very good. As each cube of meat was rescued from the pot it was greeted with a choice of five different dipping sauces on our plates.

Stabbing and cooking meat until we could hold no more we then were ushered back into the kitchen to indulge in the final course. A steaming pot of chocolate combined with a hint of rum and orange flavoring awaited us. Platters of fresh fruit, homemade gourmet marshmallows and fresh baked pound cake called to us, begging to be dipped into the dark sensuous chocolate. We needed no further prodding although our stomachs began to protest in earnest.

We toasted to the successes of some and empathized with the struggles of others and in the end, we left as better friends than when we had arrived. It has been said that a joy shared with a friend is doubled and a burden shared is reduced by half. I believe that is true. None of us were there by a false sense of motivation or obligation. None harbored a secret agenda (at least none that I know of), we were just friends. Out of the 10 friends sharing a communal meal we were vastly different and yet very much the same. Our careers are incredibly different, we have different political ideals, we have vastly different backgrounds and we probably all have different dreams and goals for the future. Yet we all have a genuine sense of caring and interest in each other.

Left to our own devices we likely would have never met. Whether by chance or fate or a preordained series of events, our lives crossed and we all became friends. Life gives us twists and turns in the road with a thousand surprises if we would only open our hearts and our eyes and enjoy the ride.

We left that evening feeling very satisfied. The food was delicious but that wasn't the important part of the meal. The best part was how we ate together. Talking and laughing and eating our evening sped by. Four and half hours later we drove away feeling very satisfied. Not wealthy from a bank account but rich from having a chorus of friends that will hug and laugh and cry and feed us in spite of really knowing us. That is truly feeling wealthy.

Grace in the Kitchen

Sharing kitchen duties is common for many married couples. The traditional nuclear family with a dog and 2 ½ children is becoming less mainstream. The wife smiling, in a cute little dress, dutifully waiting at the door for her husband to arrive home from work is a fable from the 1950's. While some may recall those images with pleasant memories, it usually isn't the wife. Now, more often than not, the first one home after a busy day is the one to start supper, and sometimes it is the child.

In my experience, those without children seem to have the best or most advice on how children should be raised. It is the same with cooking. Those with the fewest cooking skills are often the most critical and that is why having the ability to prepare decent food is something everyone should acquire. I have heard women state with absolute certainty that if they were to leave for an extended time, their beloved husbands would likely starve to death lying next to a pantry full of food. I actually have my doubts that anyone would starve, more likely he would eat plenty of toast and frozen pizza. Maybe if he was motivated the menu might include fried eggs or cereal and milk.

I have prepared my share of the food we have eaten over the years but somehow, I have fallen into a niche of making Saturday morning breakfast and coffee. It has become my accepted position of making the coffee every day and often I will make breakfast for my wife on work days as well. Saturdays, the meals tend to be a bit more involved because I have the time. More often than not I have been making a baked pancake, so simple even I can make it. Combined with natural northern Wisconsin maple syrup, a steaming mug of black coffee and some sausages or strips of bacon, it is a fitting way to start the weekend.

I prefer to have my bacon slightly on the limp side but she would rather have it so crispy that it crumbles. It is hard to compromise on something of this importance. Usually I will serve it my way and she has to live with it. This was a problem last week.

The cast iron skillet was a temptation too great for her to ignore. Rather than simply accepting the bacon the way it should be served, she turned the burner back on and commenced to char her strips of bacon. When she was satisfied with the way she thought it should be served we finished our early morning dining experience and went about our activities.

It wasn't until later in the day I reentered the house to the smell of smoke. As any homeowner knows, the smell of something burning within the house is generally to be avoided. The smoke alarm hadn't sounded and that wasn't so reassuring either. I found the cause, a bit of cremated bacon, eternally bonded to the bottom of a smoking cast iron frying pan. For a brief moment I thought I was in trouble but then I clearly recalled the additional cooking time required by my dining partner. Rather than confront her on the neglectful, forgetful, dangerous activities she participates in, I decided to hold it in reserve for the next domestic discussion.

The next day I was up with the chickens and set about my coffee making duties. We have a coffee maker that will grind the beans and brew the coffee so you always have the best coffee available to the civilized world. The machine grinds the beans which fall into a filter basket. The heated water drips into the basket and percolates through into the pot. One of the great simple pleasures of life, only this time I failed to put the coffee filter into the allotted place.

The beans ground, the water heated and I decided to spend my waiting moments out on the deck breathing in some of the freshest air of the day. Returning to the kitchen to serve myself the first cup, I was greeted with a steaming mess, coffee grounds and hot water all over the counter and down the front of the cabinets and onto the floor. Water tends to seep into cracks and each of the drawers below had collected its share of the mess.

I hurried to clean the mess but after 20 minutes of mopping and wiping my wife caught me red handed. I reasoned that if I could get this cleaned up without her knowing, I would still have her burnt frying pan as ammunition. Now that I was found to be guilty as well, I had no option other than keeping my mouth shut. And with my cooking abilities maybe that isn't a bad idea. In the kitchen, the best approach is simple; he who is without mistakes can throw the first pancake.

Cheap Dates

Profound changes occur as we march through our allotted years on this earth, many of them humbling. Just as most of us are regaining some level of sanity from our child rearing days, gravity begins an all-out assault on our bodies. One night you go to bed in fine physical shape and in the morning, you realize that you are no longer the perfect human specimen. Skin that was once taut, now sags and joints that were loose are now rusty.

Tight jeans are traded in for comfort fit stretch pants, tank tops become muffin tops and the best shoes you can wear are bedroom slippers because they don't hurt your bunions. However not everything that happens is bad or even unwanted. It is a liberating day when you begin buying clothes for comfort rather than style. Obviously, it is nice to have both but when you must prioritize, comfort wins the battle 90% of the time.

I was faced with the stark realization of the passage of time, this Thanksgiving holiday, while participating in a family discussion. One of my children announced how nice it was to finally get past the stage in her life when she didn't feel as though she had to impress anyone. It wasn't as if she didn't care, but she had arrived at the level of maturity when you can say with certainty "I am what I am" and "It is what it is". I later confided in my wife regarding my thoughts on the subject. "I am never going to be any better than I am right now". Now that is a sobering thought.

When you come to this realization, it is much easier to justify cheap dates. After 40 years of marriage and still being madly in love, (I think she feels the same way), we are inextricably joined at the wallet. That doesn't mean we don't enjoy some of the finer things in life but there is something comforting in simple living and simple choices.

Our first date ever was an afternoon enjoying the hustle and bustle of the central Burnett county fair. This was before the internet and cell phones, so we actually spent the afternoon talking rather than sending text messages to each other from across the picnic table. It is amazing what you learn about someone else when you meet face to face. When that first cheap date worked out, we tried sending real letters to each other.

Over the years we have continued to enjoy each other's companionship without the need for spending. One of my favorite cheap dates is a lazy canoe ride down one of the local rivers. No harm in bringing the fishing rod along either. Hamburgers on the grill and a cold drink on the deck for dinner is also a great dining experience and a wonderful way to unwind after work.

Since our children have become fully fledged and flew the nest we have more evening time to spend on the things we enjoy rather than parent-teacher conferences. In the spring and summer, we might be boating or casting for smallmouth bass on the river. Bowhunting fills out our fall dating schedule. Too often I am working so she leaves me behind and spends a quiet couple of hours alone but when I have some time off, she takes me along. A few weeks ago, she returned home later in the evening excited about all of the deer along the roads. We grabbed a spotlight and headed out shining for deer in the local fields. If I ignore the cost of the latest archery equipment, hunting clothes, blinds, stands and license costs, it is a cheap date. I guess you could still call it a cheap date even when she is 200 yards away and we aren't actually talking.

My advice is simple for young couples considering a long-term commitment. Take each other on a cheap date. If it works out, do it again. The odds are good you will have a happy life together. So often we focus on the most expensive, the best, the right time, the latest and greatest whiz-bang gizmo and we lose sight of the most important part of any relationship, the people. The strongest marriages are those who worked through adversity together, when everything wasn't always easy and the time wasn't always right. One of those secrets of success...Cheap Dates.

Communications 101

There is a rhetorical question that bears repeating. "If a man says something and his wife doesn't hear him, is he still wrong?" I don't know the origin of this and I can't take the credit but the answer is obvious. It became all the more apparent when faced with a recent college survey.

I learn things from my children all of the time. When they were small they would repeat in public what was said in private and I learned valuable lessons. Children tell the truth. I also learned not to fight the little battles and everything would naturally work out. If a child hates eating peas, there isn't anything you can do to alter their taste buds. They may relish the dog food and eat dirt but you won't get them to eat real food no matter how hard you try.

As they get older you quickly learn that you don't have all of the answers even if you pretend that you do. Each of our four daughters are learning to function and adapt on a professional level in different areas of expertise. Two of them challenge me with questions and observations in the health care field. One continually out performs me in the writing arena and our youngest seeks to understand how we communicate effectively not only on a social level but on the personal level.

One of her college projects obviously had to do with communication in marriage. Simultaneously she sent us a question that has consequences no matter how you answer. "How happy are you with your marriage?" The answer had to be quantified as a percentage.

You can see the obvious conundrum I was facing. If I answered 100% my wife would know that I was lying. No one is happy 100% of the time. However, if I answered somewhat less than 100% I would have to face the equally delicate question about the areas of which I wasn't happy. 50% seemed much too low but I did consider about 80% being a reasonable answer but this still left me defending my position, a situation I would rather avoid. 90% seemed a better choice but that still left me 10% unhappy.

I was cognizant of the fact that my wife was also answering the very same question at the same time. No matter what I answered I knew it had to nearly match her answer as well. Not only did I have to try and quantify my level of happiness but I also had to figure out how happy she might feel and not just this moment in time but also over the past 35 years. I knew that an inappropriate answer would likely impact her short-term happiness quotient and in turn, mine as well.

The timing of the question was fortunate as we were experiencing a lazy relaxing sort of day. I am certain that a bad day would have influenced our decisions. I pondered a bit more and punched in the answer on my phone, irretrievably sending my quantified level of marital happiness. My answer complete, I looked over at my wife to try and determine her level of happiness. She wouldn't tell me.

My phone soon buzzed with a return message. "Ha-ha Dad! Mom is happier than you are! What's wrong with you?" I was stunned. I figured that I had the perfect answer. The only logical answer that wouldn't result in trying to defend my position was 99%. She had answered 99.99%. I think she was lying.

Cutting the Cord

For many fathers, the longest walk is that final slow-motion shuffle from the back of the church to the front with your little girl hanging on to your arm. For a few more minutes or possibly until the invoice for the reception is finally paid she is yours. The problem isn't actually hanging on for one more hug, one more dance or one more hand out; the real problem is letting go.

Figuratively speaking we talk about cutting the apron strings. For those of us in the medical sciences it is sometimes easier to cut the cord, the umbilical cord. However, you decide to illustrate the process, the result should be the same. Independence is the goal we all want for our children but achieving this goal is not an easy course.

I look back on my own transition from dependent to independent and it wasn't all wine and roses. They gave me ten bucks and a one-way ticket and said "don't let the door hit you on the way out." Actually, it wasn't really this way. I didn't get the ten bucks or the ticket. Sounds cold hearted? Not really.

One of my greatest fears is not preparing my children for the inevitable challenges they will face. If they are unable to think clearly and plan accordingly then there is a good chance I have failed, not them. Sometimes this is a tough choice for parents. My own father told me that his father taught him how to swim by taking him out in boat and throwing him overboard. I doubt it happened that way. Knowing him, it is more likely they threw him off a bridge. Either way it worked.

When our children were in those formative years, those years when parents actually had some influence we made a conscious decision to set goals for our kids. Not those unrealistic parental goals of producing an Olympic athlete or an NFL all-pro linebacker. We focused on something attainable and much more meaningful. We made a specific statement of wanting to raise independent, free thinking, capable adults that would be able to face troubles and not wilt under pressure.

There is a huge risk in doing so but the reward is so much greater. The may pierce something that would cause me to cringe or they may get a tattoo somewhere or eat or drink or go places that I would not likely choose but that's the way it is. And if they finally capture whatever prize they are chasing then it isn't because I have paved the way and paid for the gas to get there.

When I walked Abby down the aisle I didn't stop to feel sorry for myself in what I might be losing because in reality she wasn't mine to keep anyway. She left home years before and went to New Zealand for a year as a 16-year-old starry eye girl. She came back a young woman. She cut those apron strings on her own and stretched her wings. I looked down at her as we stepped into the aisle leading to the front of the wedding ceremony and she smiled as she looked back at me. As much as I wanted to hang on tight and never let go, I simply guided her forward to the next exciting stage of her life. "Enjoy the moment" was the only advice I could muster. She squeezed my arm and we seemed to move effortlessly through the maze of people.

As we neared the front of the ceremony her husband-to-be smiled. He wasn't looking at me. With my final official act as father completed I handed her over to be married and gave the groom a high five. The cord was cut and she wasn't coming back. I let her go.

Is cutting the cord easy? Not a chance. But leaving the apron strings intact is far worse and will haunt you for the rest of your life. As the young couple went about the ceremony and the reception as confident adults I sat back and smiled. It was time for me to fade into the shadows just a bit in her life and let them take the reins.

The announcement came for the father-daughter dance and I got to hold her once more. We stumbled and laughed and moved our feet the wrong way at the wrong time but it didn't matter anymore. We did spins and twists and a couple of moves called "the pretzel" and it worked. I realized the apron strings may have been cut but she still has the strings to my heart.

Dance of the Mayfly

I went to the dance tonight. I didn't intend to join the party; I only went as an observer. It started out a bit slow which was fine with me because I was tired from a long day. The daytime orchestra was just winding down about the time my own supper was finished and I was able to sit back and enjoy the evening music. All day the chorus of orioles accompanied by the background of twittering finches, whirring blackbirds, buzzing hummingbirds and an occasional mournful whistle of the loon across the lake set the background for the evening dance.

Somewhere behind me a woodpecker joined the percussion section with a rapid beat which was somehow not out of character with the other more sedate participants. Below me in the lake I could hear the harrumphing and croaking of some of the evening musicians as they warmed up for the evening performance. The concert was certain to be good.

As I was waiting for the evening dance routine I was accosted by a band of rowdy hummingbirds. Magazine covers may show a crowd of hummingbirds quietly relaxed around a bowl of nectar but this is pure propaganda. There must be an adult beverage in the bowl to allow them to sit and converse, like old friends around a campfire. Not at my house. It doesn't work that way up here in the north woods. Here the hummingbirds take a quick slurp and then fly about like fighter pilots defending their right to take another slurp. It is not uncommon to have four or five hummingbirds deftly dipping and dodging in the air currents trying to avoid being skewered by their friends and no one is drinking the nectar. With friends like that, who needs enemies.

As the sun retraced its course behind the horizon the mayflies began their ritual. First there was a few, then hundreds and as the sun set we were witnesses to perhaps millions of mayflies dancing along the lakeshore. A loon called in the distance as the western sky provided a glowing orange backdrop to the scene. The clouds of mayflies fluttered frantically skyward only to stall their engines and drift downward. Up and down hundreds of times the mayflies fluttered until they were spent with no more energy to continue. Some rested on the decks, boats and shoreline but many were welcomed by the thousands of fish below. Countless circles in the mirrored lake surface revealed the growing feeding frenzy of the fish.

I tend to ruin a good story with science so bear with me. Mayflies are fascinating. Great clouds of these insects have hatched where they have been visible to Doppler weather radars. Mayflies don't have a long life in which to ponder their dreams. For them it is literally a one-shot deal. Hatched in the calm water enlightened by the setting sun they rise to the surface. Those that aren't eaten by the millions of eager fish simply fly off the surface of the water and dance in the evening air until they die. No chance to eat anything or taste the plants and waters from where they came. No chance to sing in the morning sunrise. No chances to lie about and bask in the warm afternoon sun. No abilities to fly about and explore the world around them. They don't even have functioning mouths to feed even if they wanted to. Their assigned job in the wonderful world in which we live is quite simple and spectacular.

In Asian cultures, mayflies symbolize peace, purity, prosperity and joy. It is amazing that something so simple and whose lifespan is so brief could inspire such depth of character. Hatched in the setting sun they simply reproduce and then dance until they drop. In the briefest of lives they reflect the pure joy of living by unbridled exuberance. No matter how brief your time on this earth, make sure you dance when you have the chance. Remember the mayfly.

Dining on the Edge

Dining outside of the normal safe and well equipped American kitchen can be intimidating and even dangerous. We have read about problems of contaminated food from unhealthy sources which can obviously cause health related problems. We are told to wash our hands and properly care for our food during the preparation process in order to prevent or at least reduce the risk of health problems secondary to our diet. Yet, despite taking careful precautions, sometimes it is the unexpected that will cause the greatest risk.

It has often been said, "Don't drink the water" when traveling within the borders of a foreign country but what about the food? Which food can be eaten and which should be avoided? That which looks appetizing isn't always what it seems. We attended an open-air eating experience on an island off the coast of Thailand and I avoided the steamed mussels but my adventuresome wife decided to partake, much to her chagrin. The rest of us enjoyed a delightful weekend frolicking in the coastal waters and eating in pleasant uncrowded restaurants along the coast while she curled up in bed, her moaning accompanied only by the rumblings of her inward music. She survived but vowed never to eat anything that is a degree cooler than a nuclear meltdown.

We also had a dining experience in Duluth, MN where we enjoyed four courses of wonderful food at the expense of a friend. I still consider him a friend despite the outcome. The hour was late and we decided to spend the night in a motel near Canal Park in Duluth. It was a fantastic meal and certainly no reason to complain was ever discovered during the course of our dining experience. At the hour of 3am we both spontaneously erupted from our bed. She made it to the bathroom; I only made it as far as the trash can. We spent the next 4 hours changing places. We haven't eaten there since although I haven't heard of anyone else who have entered the gates of eternity from ordering off the menu, so we may consider returning in the future. I pitied the housekeeping staff that had to clean the motel room.

Recently we had another gustatory challenge that warrants at least an honorable mention. Christmas shopping combined with a trip to view the Christmas lights in Duluth with part of our family, found us looking for a place that could handle a group of ten. We finally decided on a Japanese Hibachi type of restaurant where the grill master performs death defying acts while slicing, chopping and grilling your order in front of your very eyes.

Seated around the large hot grill we ordered drinks and sushi while the Hibachi chef did his pregame warm up. A small flood of oil on the grill along with a match and we had a cloud of flame meant to entertain and inspire us. Most of us cheered while one grandchild cowered in the corner with a healthy respect of the fire. Then came the obligatory chopping of the food while tossing a fragment for each guest to catch in their mouth. Most were successful in gulping the bite from the air; but that which was missed was probably swept up for the next day's stir fry.

The juggling portion of the chef's dining preparation show was next. He clanked the tips of his sharpened meat fork and spatula together as he flipped and twirled each instrument over the hot grill. Flip, twist, spin, twirl, clank them together and repeat. I was impressed that so much action could go into the simple process of cutting and frying onions. Cutting the onion into slices then separating them into rings, he stacked each ring into the shape of a miniature volcano. With the deft twist of his wrist he squirted some oil into the stack of onion rings and they ignited into a flash of flame and a shooting spiral of steam from the miniature Mt Vesuvius formed by onion slices on the grill in front of us.

Satisfied with his audience participation he commenced to flipping the sharp metal spatula between the dagger shaped tines of his fork. Flip, twist, clang, clack he went until all of a sudden, the spatula struck out on its own accord. Sailing out of his grasp and straight toward my wife, the flight of the sharp instrument was interrupted by her beverage glass. Just a scant few inches from her face the glass erupted into a shower of fractured glass and along with the contents, sprayed across the table and the side of the grill where she was positioned.

Surprising to me, the staff appeared from nowhere with a well-rehearsed and prompt emergency response. Drinks were mopped up, glass fragments were quickly swept away and dishes were replaced as the show progressed, as if this was a common occurrence or at least something to be expected. The rest of the chef's antics were decidedly subdued and we did finish the meal without any serious injuries or casualties

We have eaten at many places and many different food selections that have caused me to ponder the risk. In the past only the mussels or the squid has tried to kill us but this is the first time we survived an attempt on our lives directly from the chef. At least it keeps us from getting fat.

Déjà vu, All Over Again

After many years of marriage, celebrating an anniversary has become a bit easier. We celebrated with grilled chicken, fresh green beans from the garden and a quiet dinner at home. For after dinner excitement she wanted to go fishing. It took me 35 years to train her so I wasn't going to waste the opportunity. A very warm day, we bobbed around on the lake looking for fish while enjoying the sunset. It was relaxing and lazy.

The fish were lazy as well, nibbling but not biting. Sitting back in our seats we relaxed and enjoyed the sunset. It was amazing how fast the years had passed. I remember thinking that if I had it all to do over I don't think I would do anything differently. Some decisions didn't go as well as I had hoped but in the end, it worked out well. We learned, we adjusted and sometimes we just made the best out of a difficult situation. Life is like that.

Failing to catch fish in one spot we motored to another and dropped anchor. Lowering our lines, we promptly had bites. Bobbers bobbed, rods bounced and finally we caught a single fish. I unhooked it and he was quickly returned to his watery home. It was then that we heard a shout for help. At first thinking it was some swimmers across the lake we didn't respond. Then we heard it again. Looking toward the source of the sound, we saw a lone boat sitting quietly in the middle of the lake. One of the passengers waved an orange flag hoping to get our attention. The only other boat on the lake we pulled our anchor and motored toward the stranded boat. The sun had set and in the gathering darkness we identified three young people in the lake without a paddle.

"You saved our lives!" In no immediate danger, they were just stranded but happy for the assistance. "Our boat quit and the battery is dead, can you tow us to our cabin?"

"No problem" I replied and tossed them a rope as I secured the other end to my boat. We started out slowly across the lake.

"Do you know where my cabin is?" one of the boys yelled so I could hear him about the noise of the outboard motor. "It's over there." He pointed toward the opposite shore.

It was then that a sudden thought occurred to me. "Are you Charlie?" I looked back at the young man who had tied the rope to the front of his boat. He was tall and strong with a happy smile. "How did you know?" He was surprised that I had guessed his name.

"This is the second time I saved your life." He paused. I told him my name. The first time I saw Charlie was in the emergency room 15 years ago. He was an active boy who had disappeared along the lake. Two-year-old boys should be seen and heard, he was neither. A frantic search by his family led to his lifeless body submerged in the water. After CPR and emergency care he arrived in the hospital still not breathing on his own.

The first time I had ever dealt with a child drowning victim it was as if I was seeing my own child lying helpless before me. I fought to suppress my own fears and anxieties. As calmly as possible the entire ER team responded and we did what we had been trained to do all the while silently praying and hoping that what we were doing was going to be enough. A tube was inserted into his airway, IV's were started and the helicopter arrived on schedule to whisk him off to Children's Hospital.

Sometimes in life, you wonder if what you do makes a difference. You wonder if anyone really cares. You lie awake at night second guessing your own decisions, wondering if you made the right ones. Years of education and practice sometimes seems so inadequate. I looked at Charlie in the boat, strong and healthy, tanned and happy. Sometimes we do make a difference.

I asked him before we left, "Do you remember anything about that day 15 years ago?" He didn't which was just as well. I did. In a very brief moment in time it made me realize how precious life really is. He had a second chance at life and for a short moment tonight it was Déjà vu, all over again.

Dances with Loons

Vacations or holidays are by nature different from everyday life. By definition a vacation implies that we leave or vacate our normal humdrum existence and experience something out of the ordinary, something different. Sometimes we call it "R & R" meaning rest and relaxation. If that is your purpose then many such vacations can fit the bill. But a truly great holiday reaches past the boredom of day to day life and it lifts us up and inspires us. It gives us a cause and a purpose. It helps us to mix a bit of spice into our daily bland routine.

I have friends who spend their vacations building homes for less fortunate families in Mexico. They leave their own comfortable homes and drive thousands of miles, at their own expense, to work in scorching heat with limited resources and they return refreshed and inspired. I know others who take a few days off from their usual work routine and simply relax by the lake, catching up on a good book or spend some lazy hours in the garden or on a brisk walk through the countryside. Each in their own way is refreshed and inspired.

I am inspired in many ways. A golden sunset, a good book, simple food shared with friends, peace and tranquility, a quiet canoe ride down a wild river and history made alive. I like history and I think we would all be better off as history students because it has much to teach us. However, what was once old is somehow made new and can be inspiring. Our grand circle tour around Lake Superior was filled with old cities, old forts, and old rocky shorelines and each time I relive the experience, it becomes new again. I want to believe that I have learned something in the process.

Old Fort William is such a place. Perched on the Kaministaquia River on the outskirts of modern Thunder Bay, Ontario it was a vital link in the early fur trade of North America. It was the largest fur trading post and the primary intersection of traders coming out of Montreal, Quebec and the multitude of smaller outposts extended throughout Canada and northern United States. If you go to their historic maps dating back more than 200 years you can find our own Fort Folle Avoine (near Webster Wisconsin) as one of the outposts of the Northwest Company. What makes Old Fort William interesting is how the operation of the fort is displayed in living history.

Traders, merchants, cooks, blacksmiths, Natives, tin smiths, farmers and canoe makers live out their days within the confines of the fort as if it were 1812. Bread and fowl alike are roasted and baked over wood fires. No snaps, Velcro or zippers, all clothing is held in place with simple buttons, straps and buckles. Partners of the Northwest Company are seen holding meetings with clerks and traders adorned in tall black beaver hats while Natives and voyageurs are resigned to outer regions of the fort, residing canvas tents or bark wigwams. The smell of wood fires and the bleat of goats and the cluck of chickens take us all back to a simpler time.

Numerous hand-hewn log structures dot the confines of the fort. I was impressed with the fur buildings holding countless numbers of fox and beaver and other furs to be made into 90-pound packs. However most inspiring to me was the canoe shed. A large open building, it held many birch bark canoes in various stages of completeness. These birch bark canoes ranged from a simple one-person size to large freight canoes exceeding 30 feet in length with a capacity to carry 8 paddlers and 3000 pounds of cargo. Built entirely by hand out of materials available in the forest they are a testament to the ingenuity and resourcefulness of the Ojibway and the European craftsmen of that day. It was during my time in the canoe shed that I was inspired to restore something from my own past.

After leaving Thunder Bay we passed the border patrol and entered back into northern Minnesota. Through each and every state park we camped and hiked I couldn't get the canoe idea out of my head.

Nearly 22 years have passed since I built my own canoe out of cedar strips. Pieced together in my garage, it began to take shape in March of 1992 and was finally finished in the first week of November of that same year. The maiden voyage came as skim ice was forming on the shores of our lake. In celebration of getting her parking space back in the garage, my wife bought me a hand-crafted paddle made of the finest wood and had the same deep red-brown coloration as the newly completed canoe. "Dances with Wolves" was one of the most popular movies of that time and so I borrowed the theme and had a brass plate engraved. It was mounted on the bow with the words "Dances with Loons 1992"

That canoe was my friend and companion in many trips down our wild rivers and also into Boundary Waters in northern Minnesota. It was on one of these trips that my canoe became intimate with a large rock and the hull was cracked. For years since that infamous meeting it has hung in solitude, perched beneath the rafters of my shed. Through my own neglect and indifference, it became checked and weathered and fell into further states of disrepair.

History lessons have a way of reminding us of our own history. Upon our return home from the craggy shores of Lake Superior, I promptly removed the old cedar strip canoe from the rafters and swept out the dust of history. I smiled as I recalled the good times. I ran my hand over the cracked hull and the water stained wood. With inspiration from the past I began the repair process to restore the old canoe to its former glory. With some hard work it will again resume its rightful place on the wild waters and live up to its name, "Dances with Loons".

Vacations don't have to be exotic or expensive. You don't have to fly away to distant lands and eat strange food. You don't need to spend a worldly fortune to have a world class experience. Sometimes the greatest holiday is in our own backyard. To rest, relax and be restored is enough, but to be inspired is icing on the cake. If you want to find a bit of everything, try driving in circles. Take the greatest circle of all around Lake Superior, you will be inspired.

Keyed Up

"**Where** did you put my keys?"

"What keys?"

"My truck keys, I put them right here so I wouldn't lose them. What did you do with them?"

"Why would I do anything with your keys?" She resisted the overpowering urge to roll her eyes in frustration. "Why didn't you put them somewhere safe?" We were in the last evening of a fly-in Canadian fishing trip. The float plane was due to arrive at 7:30 in the morning to fly us back to civilization where we would load up our truck and head back across the border toward home. Bags were packed, fishing gear stowed and last-minute preparations were in place so we could depart efficiently in the morning. My only concern was no car keys.

"Are you sure you put them here?" She searched through the top, middle and bottom drawers of the small dresser in the remote cabin. Nothing remained to be seen but she began to sense my desperation and pulled each drawer out and checked and rechecked and then checked again. No keys.

With anything misplaced, which seems to happen all too often at this stage of my life, I did my best to retrace my steps and rethink every action I had completed since I had last handled the keys. Over the past 4 days I got in the boat and went fishing, got out of the boat and ate too much, got into the boat and went fishing, got out of the boat and ate more and then went to bed. The next day I repeated my steps except I was bundled into five layers of clothes to ward off the wind and rain and cold. The 3rd and 4th days were mirror images of the first two. If the keys weren't where I had placed them then I must have put them into a jacket pocket for safe keeping.

Bags carefully packed for the flight out were torn asunder in frantic attempts to search each and every pocket and wrinkle. I discovered my rain gear and jackets had somewhere around 30 different pockets all protected by zippers and Velcro. I went through each crevice with growing fear of hitching hiking across the International border. No keys. My fishing tackle bags were opened and reopened again without results. I discovered old pliers, knives, bug spray and a petrified tube of lip balm but no car keys. I glanced at the clock, only 10 hours until the float plane arrived. Time was short.

"You must have put them somewhere else, you always do that and then you don't remember what you did with them." I could sense her growing anxiety as she returned to the small dresser for the 4th time. She searched under the bed, in the corners and the bathroom with a small flashlight but still no keys. To make matters worse she caught an earring and flipped it out onto the floor. (Yes, she is a classy angler and she fishes with diamond earrings). I wasn't exactly feeling compassionate about a lost earring when we would be spending the winter in Ft. Francis Ontario because we had no transportation. If we didn't find the keys we could at least pawn her remaining earring and get a taxi ride across the river. Then maybe we could contact a friend or relative to come and get us. Funny things run through your mind in times of desperation. I realized most of our relatives would probably leave us there.

"It must have been some kids that came in and took my keys." I thought to myself, but we were 150 miles from any kids. It is always good to have some kids around to take the blame. My stomach acid was increasing in strength. A dose of antacids would likely help me to refocus. Digging through my shaving kit suddenly before my eyes my keys appeared. "When did you put my keys in here?"

"Why would I do that? That is your stuff not mine." She paused to let her blood pressure ease out of dangerous range. "I can't believe it, you do this every time!"

The float plane arrived on time and we had an uneventful flight back to civilization. We loaded our truck and began to cross the river toward the USA border station.

I offered a simple apology. "Sorry about the keys, I am glad we found them and your earring. Over all I had a good time." She nodded in agreement. All's well that ends well.

"I just have one more question." She turned to me with concern in her eyes. "What did we do with our passports?"

Last Week

There is an oft repeated phrase that applies to vacations and vacationer everywhere; "You should have been here last week!" Implying that whatever you are doing, no matter where you are and whatever the weather, it was always near perfection last week or yesterday or whenever you weren't there.

With us it is nearly always the case. I have traveled all over the world and one of the first things I am told by the local residents is "This is very unusual weather, you should have been here last week." One past June, several years ago, we traveled to western Alberta, Canada, to the town of Banff. Tammy proudly explained to our entire family how beautiful the alpine flowers are along the hiking trails leading to Peyto Lake, a popular destination in the area. We drove with anticipation to the parking area leading to the lookout viewing area above the lake. Pulling into the parking area it became apparent that our expectations needed to be amended. The snow banks surrounding the parking area were taller than our car. We couldn't see the flowers along the trail because they were buried in knee deep snow in late June. Our family photo standing on the viewing platform shows our children huddled behind winter coats with upturned collars to shield themselves from the biting wind and stinging ice pellets in the air. We were told by everyone how beautiful is normally is and we should have been there last year. Typical.

Finally, I can say with a sense of satisfaction, I was on vacation last week, not only in a literal sense but in the figurative sense as well. For once, nearly everything went well. My wife, my daughter Leah and her husband John and myself traveled together to a remote fishing resort in northwestern Ontario, Canada called Moose Point Lodge. To reach that location you have to travel by float plane about 140 miles from the international border at International Falls, MN. I envisioned mechanical problems, weather problems and a confused pilot. None of these came true. In fact, the plane was on time and the weather was cooperative. The pilot was friendly and even allowed my son-in-law to sit in the copilot seat, not because he has any flying experience but he had the longest legs and while we were huddled in cramped seating arrangements in the luggage department, he rode in style.

We landed at the resort on time and breakfast was ready, hot steaming pancakes, mugs of strong black coffee, slabs of homemade bread with blueberry jam, eggs any style you wanted, all served by friendly faces and happy people. I pinched myself. It normally doesn't work that way for me. While we stuffed our faces with a fantastic breakfast our luggage and fishing gear was delivered to our cabin intact, nothing lost or broken.

Following breakfast, we went fishing and believe it or not, we caught fish, so many fish that our arms ached and we looked forward to long boat rides so we could rest our tired backs and shoulders. Lunch was served on rustic tables along the shore, crispy fried potatoes, onions, beans and heaps of browned walleye fillets, cooked to perfection. My only mishap was burning my mouth on a bite of fish hot from the frying pan.

The first evening we returned to the lodge where mountains of lasagna dripping with tomato sauce and cheese were placed on our plates. We didn't leave the table hungry that night or any night. Each and every day we repeated the script, eating, fishing, laughing, eating, fishing, telling stories, eating... On the final day it was cool and cloudy with a chance of rain. After a near perfect week we figured we could handle a bit of adversity. Prepared for inclement weather we spent the morning searching for cooperative fish. As noon approached, the clouds parted and the sun shone bright on our shore lunch picnic spot. Even the insects, normally intent on inflicting injury to unsuspecting visitors were surprisingly docile.

On the final day as we departed the resort on our float plane escort out of the wilderness I overheard new guests inquiring about the fishing success. Our fishing guide smiled, "The fishing is always good, but you should have been here last week." For five wonderful days God smiled on our party and we smiled back. It was last week and we were there.

Life's a Butter Dream

It seems as though summer escaped our detection this year. One moment I was relaxing with the anticipation of a sunny summer day and the next I realized I missed it. Our home is in transition at the moment. One child moved out and another moved back accompanied by her family. The hustle and bustle of the transition to a new school year is now fully in place. What was once a past experience has now returned to our home front. We can now delight in our grandchildren challenging their own parents about school lunches, school clothes and school activities. What hasn't changed is the sudden passing of summer into fall. I pulled up an old story from a couple of years ago because it captures the mood quite well.

Summertime, sweet summertime, while not my favorite season, it certainly ranks in the top four. Summer is the season for adventure. Plans, written and reviewed through the winter and spring are brought to fruition during that glorious season known as summer. Summer is the season for fun. Baseball games, picnics and back yard campouts fill our free time as work and other priorities get pushed into tomorrow. Summertime is the time to relax and enjoy some of the fruits of your work. There is something very satisfying about relaxing in the shade with cold drinks, friends and no schedule to interrupt your thoughts.

Summer is also a mad dash to the finish. Life here in the upper Midwest seems to leap from season to season with such quickness that it leaves us little time to think. It seems that as soon as we finish putting the snow shovels away, we look around and realize that the maple leaves are starting to turn red. Life becomes a blur as we try to take it all in.

I am not an advocate for laziness but if I had to choose between that and busyness, I would lean toward the first every time. Laziness however implies a definite tendency toward willful avoidance of work and that is not generally considered a good choice. Perhaps a better way would be unscheduled time and a slower pace of living. Unscheduled time allows us to respond to the need or opportunity of the moment. If neighbors or friends suddenly have an overabundance of brats or burgers on their grill, who among us wouldn't like to be able to respond and assist them in their time of need?

We just completed the final weekend of the summer and after our children left it was suddenly quiet. While filled with movement and noise it was anything but busy. It was spontaneous and fun, relaxing and fulfilling. It was an example of what summer and actually life should be. Grilling on the deck turned into hours of relaxed conversation as we talked about anything and everything. Later that evening, in our living room we somehow transitioned into a spontaneous display of talent or lack of talent and then family games. Never was anything planned, but rather it happened as we allowed it to happen in a relaxed and supportive environment. Nearly the entire weekend we laughed and ate and relaxed together and nothing was planned except for one event. The summer canoe trip.

This wasn't a planned route into the back country of Boundary Waters, nothing of the sort. This was simply a slow and lazy trip down one of the local rivers. Most years we head down the Namekagen or the St Croix rivers but this year we went in our own backyard, the Yellow River. As parents, however, we have ulterior motives with the canoe trip. We have found this to be a good judge of character. Two of our daughters were home from college with friends of the opposite sex, one of them rather serious and one not so serious but that wasn't the point. We have discovered that if they could paddle a canoe around sticks, stumps, logs and sandbars in a coordinated and cooperative manner without complaining then very likely they would be able to negotiate other speed bumps in life in the same manner.

It was a near perfect day as we drifted around tight corners in the river and watched eagles drifting high above us in the cloudless sky. Surrounded by friends, grown up children and singing grandchildren, we enjoyed a near perfect ending to the summer. We were gratified to watch them working together without serious conflict. As we neared the final destination our five-year-old granddaughter Ella, began to sing at the top of her lungs.

"Row, row, row your boat,
Gently down the stream
Merrily, merrily, merrily, merrily
Life's a butter dream."

On that particular sunny Sunday afternoon, I couldn't agree more.

Little Women

Louisa May Alcott may have the originator of the title *Little Women* but she is by no means the only one who understands little women. Her book originally published in September of 1868 chronicled the lives of 4 women as they challenged the gender constraints of their day and lived in a way that demonstrated the triumph of virtue over social position and wealth. While I cannot say I understand the thoughts and feelings of each of the women I can say with some degree of empathy, I can understand the feelings of the father.

I have been incredibly blessed and I am eternally grateful for the wonderful women in my life. And it seems as though the blessings continue. Most of you know I have four daughters and each of them has grown into their own way of life. Recently we had the chance to marry off one more, our third daughter. I have one daughter remaining on the household payroll.

It has been a recurring theme over the years that when people find out we have 4 girls and only 4 girls everyone seems to express some sympathy as if I have been cheated somehow. I can assure you, I am not cheated but rather blessed beyond any measure I could have hoped for.

"What? No boys"

"Think of the all the weddings!" Or in the words of Bill Cosby we somehow haven't figured out how to "put the stem on the apple."

At times I wonder what my life would have been like if I had a son but I quickly dismiss the thought because it really isn't worth dwelling upon. After all, my 3 oldest have not left me but rather have brought 3 wonderful sons back with them. I am thankful I have something in common with each of them and the best part is that they didn't grow up and learn all my bad habits.

Amazingly the story doesn't stop there because last week we were pleased to welcome into the world another girl, another granddaughter our 5th. That's right; we now have four daughters and five granddaughters. My life is starting to sound like a soap opera. We could have our own reality television series "9 and Counting".

Let me take a moment to introduce each of the little women including my own daughters. My challenge has been to actually memorize their names and faces and keep it all straight. If you are like me, when you want to address someone you start with a name and go through the family, your friends, a couple of pets and half of the phone book before you actually hit the right name. My list of names to remember has enough similarities between the names I am sure to mix them up from time to time.

Here is the list, Leah Beth, Anna Laura, Abigail Luray, Billie Kay, Ella Bonny, Lilyanne Hazel, Evangeline Judy,

Grace Elizabeth, Evianna Hope and now the latest edition to our family, Charlotte Emma. I also need to add my wife and matriarch of this group, Tammy Kay. Try to memorize that and repeat it backwards.

Don't worry about me. It takes a tough guy to stand up and swim against the virtual tidal wave of estrogen in my house. However, when things get tough in life it is always the girls that come to the rescue. When dear old dad or grandpa needs help one of my little girls will be sure to volunteer their husband to assist me. Maybe when I retire I will rewrite the book and entitle it *Lots of Little Women*.

Man Eating Whale

When traveling in foreign countries we try to get a real flavor for each country we visit and sampling the local foods is a great place to start. Some food items may surprise you so don't arrive with preconceived ideas. Americans have a way of labeling certain foods often from their country of origin but if you visit these countries, you may be disappointed. Italian dressing is unheard of in Italy, French dressing is scorned by the French, Canadian bacon doesn't exist north of the border and Danish pastry is a bit different than what is served here. When traveling in Thailand we were offered American fried rice. Naturally we had never heard of such a thing so we investigated. American fried rice is simply fried rice with cut up hot dogs. Apparently, Thai's have a good understanding of the American diet.

On a recent voyage to the Scandinavian countries we enjoyed visiting the local restaurants to try their offerings. First of all, we found out that Norwegians love the restaurant "TGIFridays" which is an export from the US. We found many such eating establishments on our ventures through the cities. McDonalds also seems to exist in every country around the world. Since these were clearly exports from our own country we avoided them and went to the local locations.

Dining out in Norway is not significantly different than here except you need to learn to say "Uff Da!" Not because it has anything to do with dining out, but rather it helps you to prepare for the cost. Thankfully everything was priced in Kroner so you don't really feel the impact until you get home. I could work out the conversion in my head but this required two credit cards and a calculator. I chose simply to enjoy the food and the setting and pay for it with the play money in my wallet. A sampling of prices would be as follows. Hamburger $150 NOK (Norwegian Kroner); Coke $25NOK; Shrimp dinner $180 NOK; and for you beer drinkers out there, imported beer (Budweiser) $65 NOK. Since it was all monopoly money anyway it didn't really phase us until we did the math. Six to one is the conversion so that simple cheeseburger and fries was slightly more than twenty bucks. Throw in a beverage and lunch for two was a typical $60-70 ticket. Uff Da.

One item on the menu that intrigued me was whale. I haven't seen it offered anywhere here in northern Wisconsin so at a seaside outdoor restaurant in Norway, I tried it. I was curious as to what type of whale it was but no one was sure. Obviously with beef there are different qualities of cattle such as Black Angus or Hereford or even old Holstein but apparently whales aren't categorized that way. Likewise, cattle offer differing cuts varying in quality and price. You could order a New York strip or a porterhouse or fillet mignon but not so with whales. I ordered the whale steak because when in Norway do as the Norwegians do. Actually, I didn't see anyone else in Norway eating the whale so maybe I should have stayed with TGIFridays.

Since I was investigating the local flavors, my beloved wife decided to indulge herself in the locally caught Norwegian lobster. Our tall blonde server assured us that these were fine choices, however she quickly returned to our table, inquiring about the size of the lobster required. Norwegian lobsters differ from their North American counterparts because they are priced by the gram and weighed out with gold nuggets to counterbalance the scale. I checked my supply of monopoly money and she decided a modest sized one would do just fine.

The meal was great in many ways. Unique and tasty we enjoyed it all. The lobster was served chilled with different types of sauces blended with mayonnaise that offered a distinct difference from the usual hot steaming lobster dripping with butter. The whale steak was far different than expected. I anticipated something greasy but it was very lean and deep red and was cooked medium rare to avoid toughness according to our server. I sliced off a corner and was surprise by the tenderness. The flavor however was vastly different than any land animal I had eaten, and I have tried many. I suspect it may have been similar to an old goat who had dined on garbage for years and was left to age in a warm place. I thoughtfully chewed for a minute before swallowing.

"Well...How is it?" she asked from across the table. Rather than answering I simply smiled and offered her a slice. In a nice restaurant it is hard to gag politely but she did it. The cost for our local flavors was rounded out to $1100 NOK. We had a whale of a time.

Marriage and Chemotherapy

The "Nag Factor" label was originally coined to represent the constant begging which is bombarded upon parents by their loving children in order to get what they want. Unfortunately, it seems to work by wearing the parents down to the point until they have no strength to resist and simply give in. This very same concept is now being discussed as part of a study on the effect marriage has on cancer survival. Improved survival from cancer among married couples is attributed to the "Nag Factor".

The study is actually very revealing. The Harvard study reviewed data from 750,000 individuals who had been diagnosed with the top 10 most common forms of cancer which included prostate cancer, breast cancer, colon cancer, lung cancer and others. What they found were men who were married had a 23% improved chance of survival and women had a 16% improved chance of survival over those with a similar diagnosis and treatment plan but were not married.

It seems married people tend to diagnosed in an earlier stage of the disease and are more likely to follow through on the treatment plan because married couples tend to have help remembering appointments, more likely to go to screening physical exams and have better social support during difficult times. The difference seems to be the fact that married couples encourage each other to seek appropriate medical care.

Now as much as I dislike nagging, and I really do hate nagging, I realize there can be benefits. We have been married for more than 40 years, most of it happy and I have successfully resisted any attempts at nagging. I am sure that she would never refer to repetitive suggestion making as nagging but she does help to remind me of relatively important things. About the only things in my life that don't require supervision are eating meals and perhaps outdoor recreation such as hunting, fishing, camping, boating and spending a sunny afternoon in my backyard hammock. Nearly everything else needs a reminder. Reminding me once is ok, twice is a nag.

Eight years ago, my driver's license expired and I drove all over the United States for 6 months without a valid license before it was brought to my attention. I know the State of Wisconsin DMV sent me a reminder but that wasn't enough. They didn't nag me. It was my auto insurance company that felt the need to nag me and I finally took the time to renew my license. Unfortunately, my photo was less than appealing to my wife so for the past 8 years she has been nagging me to renew my license on time so I can get a different photo that is acceptable to her way of thinking.

Unfortunately, she forgot to nag me for the past 4 months because my birthday came and went and I forgot to renew my driver's license again so I am once more driving illegally. I am relying on the good nature and forgiveness of Barney Fife until I can be formally renewed and once again safe to drive. By the time you read this I will be restored to the good graces of the State of Wisconsin.

However, I should return to the original premise of this article. With any medical study it is critical to compare the benefits as well as the risks of the different treatment options. Marriage is reported to better than chemotherapy but what about the side effects?

I can't determine what others have experienced but I can reflect on my own experience with marriage. Despite being very satisfied with our marriage, I have gained weight, I have noticed increased aching in my back and hips, I have become less inclined to participate in some activities and my hair is beginning to fall out. It sounds like the side effects are about the same.

Hidden Treasures

I love a good treasure hunt. I have often thought about the idea of searching for hidden treasures in far off lands or ancient civilizations. Lost treasures can reveal much about those who traveled this way in previous times. Who among us has not wondered about finding a secret treasure map and discovering untold fortunes? I do not own a metal detector but I have always considered the possibilities of searching old homesteads and forgotten school yards. What interesting things might be revealed? Perhaps old coins, jewelry, buttons and rusted trinkets once thought valuable but lost or discarded over time only to be rediscovered and recycled as a treasure of the discoverer.

While living on the old farm of my great grandparents I dug through the dirt and junk buried beneath the floor of the old home where my grandmother was born. Old rusted pots, nails and broken jars were dug up from the dark recesses and then I discovered a coin. It was an Indianhead penny from 1907. Back in the day when it was lost through the crack in the floor it was worth a penny but a quick check of its value today it is worth all of 98 cents in good condition. The real value to me was the fact that it was lost by my grandmother or one of her siblings or perhaps her parents over a hundred years ago. Unfortunately, I have since misplaced the same penny and it may yet be rediscovered by my own grandchildren.

It has been said that a treasure may reveal much about those who went before us. It has also been said that the garbage dumps of civilizations past reveal much more. One person's trash is another's treasure.

My daughter, home from college decided to make herself helpful. She offered to clean my truck. I use my truck. It isn't a showcase with shiny wheels, polished chrome and spotless mirrors. It is a truck that I use to haul wood, dirt and creatures both living and dead depending on the season. It can cruise down interstate highways or two rutted woodland trails with equal aplomb. It is rugged enough to tow heavy equipment but fine enough to carry my loving spouse for an evening of fine dining and entertainment.

What I didn't realize was how much of my life was accumulating in the back seat. I like to be efficient so it was not uncommon to keep an extra jacket or hat within easy reach, available for any change in the weather. Then it is always nice to have a few tools in case of emergency and perhaps a flashlight. What she discovered was something a bit more substantial.

This is what she recorded on her own Facebook page. "A truck says a lot about a man...
4 jackets, 2 pants, 2 flannel shirts, 2 pairs of shoes, 3 cans of bug spray, 9 hats, 3 pairs of gloves, a water cooler, 2 trail

cameras, coffee mug, 2 water bottles, GPS, 2 packer flags, binoculars, 2 buckets, 1 candle, tool box, 1 watch, 5 really old CDs, plenty of odds and ends and garbage, and $3.34. You're welcome dad."

I wondered what some future archeologist might surmise after sifting through the back seat of my truck. It might be decided that I was a junk dealer or perhaps I was always ready for whatever the world throws at me. Or maybe it just means the mosquitos are really bad in northern Wisconsin.

In a Rich Man's World

I have long believed that the world operates on the golden rule; those that have the gold make the rules. How many of us have spent countless hours working at our jobs, scrimping and saving something for that someday when we can relax in relative luxury, enjoying the fruits of our labors. Most of us would love to be counted as members of the privileged class, the holders of the gold. Some save and invest, some buy land and build great things, some invent or develop, some discover great wealth, some inherit and some buy lottery tickets.

Abba, the popular singing group from the 1980's, had a song entitled "Money, Money, Money". It was a lyrical story about someone who worked hard to pay bills but hoped to meet someone rich, dreaming about all the things they would do if they suddenly had money in a rich man's world. Ironically a couple from Missouri and also an unnamed person or persons from Arizona just won the national Powerball lottery. Splitting the winnings and after paying the inevitable taxes they will pocket over 132 million dollars. Not bad for a day's work. Sounds wonderful doesn't it?

Ironically winning the lottery is anything but delightful. Most lottery winners are bankrupt within five years and their lives are destroyed. Jack Whittaker, winner of the Powerball on Christmas day 2002 is just such an example. Already worth an estimated 17 million dollars at the time, he won nearly 320 million dollars with the single winning ticket. Within a few years his entire life was destroyed. Despite pledging 10 % to a Christian charity and also starting a foundation for economically disadvantaged people in West Virginia, he was robbed of hundreds of thousands of dollars after being drugged at a strip club and he lost his daughter and granddaughter to drug related deaths. Despite suddenly coming into serious wealth he wished he had torn up the winning ticket.

The story repeats itself over and over. Lottery winners are little different than many professional athletes who suddenly find themselves wealthy. Many of them have their lives destroyed and are penniless and bankrupt within 5 years. A very wise person once said, "The love of money is the root of all evil". Maybe he was right.

The lottery has been criticized as an insidious tax on the poor. The poor spend a disproportionate portion of their assets for a chance at winning. Winning may seem a dream come true but the American dream quickly becomes the American nightmare. Wealthy are far more likely to risk their cash on the stock market, real estate or even gambling, all with much higher odds of winning.

The odds of winning the Powerball lottery is about 1 chance out of 176 million. You are far more likely to be crushed by a vending machine, have identical quadruplets and die from being left handed in a right-handed world. Not very good odds no matter how you look at it.

Actor Will Smith has some very wise insight with respect to wealth. "Money and success don't change people; it only amplifies what is already there". I think he has something there. I don't consider myself above the crowd, better than anyone else. I also realize that money isn't the answer to all of our problems. But I think I am like most people believing that what I would like is a chance to prove that money doesn't buy happiness.

Old Time Medicine

Few things cause as much consternation as facing change especially when we don't really know what to expect as a result of the change. This is our situation as we are in the midst of the implementation of health care reform, whatever that may be. This isn't meant to be a political statement for or against changes in the way our medical system operates but it is meant to highlight the fact that change in any form can be challenging and difficult to accept. Last week I wrote about health care reform and this is somewhat in response to some of the comments I received.

There is an old song that has been sung in many churches across America entitled "Old Time Religion". It was likely written by someone who was frustrated or certainly concerned about the manner in which people were worshiping at church. If you take that same idea and apply it to health care reform you might come up with the concept of "Give me some of that old time medicine". So I thought that I would dig back into the history of medicine and bring up some of that old time medicine and see if we were better off.

Diabetes is an affliction that was documented as early as 1552 BC in Egypt. Although the symptoms of frequent urination were recognized it wasn't until much later that sugar was discovered as a contributing factor. Actually in 1550 Hindus recognized that ants were attracted to the urine from individuals with this affliction. However, it wasn't until the 11th century that doctors finally got the courage to taste the urine and blood of people with diabetes and it was discovered to be sweet. Since we are in the process of longing for the old-time medicine, don't expect your physicians or nurses to do any taste testing. I for one am thankful for some modern medicine.

Treatment is another matter. While diabetes could be recognized thousands of years ago, no effective treatment actually existed until the early 1900's, prior to that most people died, often with days or weeks of the onset of the disease. One of the early treatments included the "Oat Cure" which was simply a mixture of 8 ounces of oats and 8 ounces of butter. The patient was instructed to eat this every 2 hours and hope for the best. If that treatment didn't work then you could always rely on the whiskey and black coffee remedy. An equal mixture of each was also given to the patient every two hours. I am sure it was successful at reducing any pain but again no one actually survived the treatment.

Many, many years ago Hippocrates believed people were composed of blood, phlegm, yellow bile and black bile. However, since then we have discovered more than 4 basic fluids within our makeup. Cancer was thought to be due to an excess of black bile but no one really understood the process. Despite the realization of the seriousness of cancer in its many forms, few treatment options were available or effective. The Egyptians had one of the most troubling options what was described as the fire drill. While it was effective at inflicting pain and fear into the patient it was palliative at best.

The really interesting tidbits of health care come from ancient Rome. Hyena parts play a very active role in the delivery of health care at that time. It would seem that various parts of a hyena could cure nearly any known ailment. However, administration of the hyena parts needed to be handled carefully. If you apply the left foot of the hyena to a woman in labor it could have fatal consequences but application of the right foot was certain to accelerate labor and result in a successful delivery. Ambidextrous goat parts were found to lack effectiveness.

Gout was an affliction of the well-to-do as they tended to have access to the better cuts of meat such as liver and kidneys. Treatment of gout was an aromatic process. Application of cow dung and vinegar was one option however if that didn't work then a combination of goat suet and mustard or possibly ashes of goat dung combined with axel grease. Before filling your prescription, make sure to check with your pharmacist to determine which poultice is approved by your insurance carrier. Also remember that generic goat dung is generally cheaper than brand name Billy Goat dung.

Over the Top

Living with another human being is a demanding process capable of dividing even the most dedicated relationship. Major issues of mutual interest such as buying a new car, house or even moving to another state are seldom the thorn that incites the most pain. Rather it is the relatively minor areas of concern that derives the largest emotional response and thereby is the most divisive. Nothing infuriates an otherwise orderly and docile person more than squeezing the toothpaste tube in the middle when everyone should already know you squeeze it from the bottom up. Welcome to the big stuff.

Marriage has been discussed within our household on numerous occasions within the past year, largely because one of our delightful offspring is in the process of preparing for an upcoming wedding. We are also in the process of a major event at work. Discarding one form of computer software in exchange for a different way of doing things is not unlike a marriage. When discussing this process with a co-worker I presented my view as being very much similar to the wedded bliss we all seem to experience at one point or another. No one marriage is perfect and anyone going into a marriage with the idea that their spouse is perfect will be sorely disappointed because we all have our quirks. The happiest and most stable relationship is when each, with eyes wide open, sees the faults of the other and is willing to adapt and commit despite the differences.

During a brief lapse in my daily schedule I happened upon a group of co-workers deep in discussion about something of grave importance. Wondering if I was the subject of the meeting I promptly burst in on the scene. I was relieved to know that we weren't discussing issues of life and death, it was much more serious.

"How do you put the toilet paper on the holder? Does it unroll underneath or over the top?" That was the question posed to me as I arrived at the edge of the gathering. I didn't have to think much because everyone knows it goes "over the top". Someone else added a more important issue concerning the availability of the toilet paper. If you use the last of the roll, do you take the time to replace it or do you leave that dilemma to next person in line to the throne room. If you don't have any left in the immediate vicinity you had better hope your room mate will deliver some at your hour of need without taunting.

These questions got me thinking back to the time we were first married and how we adapted to the other's quirks and quibbles. I reviewed in my mind the many unasked and unanswered questions we somehow managed. Do you spend Christmas with his family or her family? Do you keep the temperature in the bedroom cool or warm? Do you wear pajamas or do you prefer to be close to the sheets? Do you wear your shoes in the house or do you skip around in socks and slippers? Do you share the same soap, shampoo and toothpaste or have your own? Do you pinch the toothpaste tube from the bottom or squeeze it in the middle? Do you leave the bathroom door open while attending to the calling of nature or do you shutter the windows, close the curtains and lock the doors?

It is said that the measure of disappointment is the difference between expectations and reality. In our marriage of over 36 years I can safely say that I am not disappointed, not because of a lack of expectations or a blind eye to reality but rather a simple gesture of humility. The first thing every morning I wake up and say I'm sorry. It helps to relieve any guilt that may accumulate during the day.

Anyway, after the discussion at work I decided to go home and find the truth about toothpaste and toilet paper. We each have our own tubes and she agrees the paper should roll out over the top. At least we agree on something.

Partly Cloudy

Living in northern Wisconsin the weather tends to be a focal point of our day to day conversations. If we aren't talking about our favorite sports teams or politics, or the price of gas, we are talking about the weather. Politics may raise our ire or stir our emotions, sports may capture our passion and our devotion but the weather or at least the forecast of the weather confuses us all.

My wife seems to be focused on the news in general. She has a need to see the 10 o'clock news before heading off to bed, even if she falls asleep on the couch 5 minutes into the program. I would rather pass on the news, as most of it seems to be depressing anyway. It is during the weather forecast, I tend to show more interest which then carries over into the sports.

We have hosted many students from other countries that to my amazement, seems to have little or no interest in the weather forecast. I have asked them if they ever check the weather forecast at home and the answer was almost never. Of course, their answers always seemed logical. In Thailand, there was no need to check the weather forecast. It was either very hot through most of the year or very hot and raining thorough the rest of the year. Apparently, meteorologists in Thailand have little chance of being wrong in the forecast.

Living in a land of four seasons, weather dominates our activities. It seems we are always wondering about the forecast or complaining that the forecast is wrong. Farmers, completely dependent on the weather, hope for adequate rain and warm temperatures at planting time and dry weather at harvest. Anglers hope for pleasant weather to be on the water but wish for low pressure before a storm front because that tends to stimulate fish activity. Young couples and the mother of the bride always pray for dry sunny weather for outdoor weddings. Yet no matter what we need or hope for, the meteorologist always seems to get it wrong, or at least different enough to make us think he or she is wrong.

I would recommend that we give up on billion-dollar radars, satellite images and computer-generated weather models. These do nothing more than give us false hope. I am not saying that the forecast is wrong; it is simply limited in its ability to deliver accurate information despite the latest technology and the tremendous cost.

I would recommend returning to the basic means of weather prediction as this is actually more accurate. Most of us have heard of the weather rock. If it is wet, it is raining; if it is hot it is sunny; if it is covered in ice, then it is cold outside etc. While being very accurate, it lacks predictability. It only tells us what is happening at that moment in time. This is ok for the city, but here in the country we need something with a longer range rather than what is happening at the moment.

Since I live close to nature as most of us do here in northern Wisconsin, I have researched natural ways of predicting the weather and I hope you are able to use them to your advantage. For instance, did you know that if a cow bellows three times in a row, a storm is not far behind? If ant hills are small it will be a hot dry summer. Did you know that if leaves drop early, Indian summer will be short and we will have a mild winter, but if the beavers put more logs and mud on the north side of the beaver lodge then it will be a hard winter. If there are skinny rabbit tracks in the snow that means a thaw is at hand unless of course,, they were just made by a skinny rabbit.

Some of the most reliable ways of predicting weather is listening to my wife. When her shoulder aches I know it is going to rain and when she has a headache it has nothing to do with the weather. When my back aches I know it is going to be nice weather because when the weather is nice I use my back ache as an excuse to avoid doing yard work and go fishing. The method I have the most problem with is crickets. It has been said that if you count up the number of cricket chirps in 14 seconds and add 40 you will arrive at the accurate temperature in Fahrenheit. If you want the temperature in Celsius then you should count the number of chirps in 8 seconds and add 4.

I tried this one evening last week. Trying to listen to just one cricket is the problem. I had several of them trying to predict the weather. Between that and the ringing in my ears I determined it was 137 degrees outside. Now that is a forecast I can believe in.

Personality Plus

Someone once described marriage as being similar to ordering a meal at a nice restaurant. You review the menu and make your selection and after the food comes you look at what everyone else got and you wish you would have ordered that. Bad analogy and bad advice. Marriage is much more complicated than that and the choices are never quite as simple as picking something out of the menu. You may be thinking about the main dish but there is often a side salad we didn't plan on.

When we first met the internet wasn't even a thought and online dating meant talking on the party line when someone else might be listening. However online dating services seem to offer something with at least a remote similarity to making a menu selection. What once seems rather strange and unnatural has now become quite common place. The basic premise is simple. You enter your information into a database and so does everyone else and the computer does all the work. Those with disparate issues are never introduced but those with similar interests and personalities are then given the chance to offer more information and eventually meet if that is their choice. You no longer have to brush your teeth and worry about bad breath until you are well along in the dating process, most of which is initially carried out in dating cyberspace.

After saying "I'm sorry" for more than 35 years, I was wondering what would happen if we both filled out anonymous personal profiles in a dating database, would we actually be compatible? Would the all-knowing powers of the internet actually link us up for eternal excitement and contented bliss? Would we be allowed the opportunity to electronically "wink" at one another before being allowed the chance to have lunch together? As interesting as it may seem retrospectively doing this may be a bad idea. First of all you might not find yourselves as compatible as you think or you may actually find out you are perfect for each other and about 17 other people. Then what?

As an alternative exercise we took a personality test which is quick and free online. 16personalities.com offers a free and simple test that will reveal your innermost thought processes with amazing clarity and astounding accuracy. It even gives you a good explanation about why your spouse is so hard to understand and also why you act the way you do.

I found out that I am extroverted, likable, quick witted and original and I like to argue. This was definitely news to me. I had always assumed it was my wife that liked to argue. She tried to agree with the report but I argued that you can't believe everything you read on the internet. I also found out that I like to brainstorm, think big and have little respect for the rules. Don't bother me with details, they are irrelevant. I would rather improvise later than plan now.

She read the report and agreed wholeheartedly with the findings. She now understood why I talk big but the lawn never gets mowed and things around the house are fixed with duct tape and a hot glue gun. Next it was my turn to review her personality profile.

I read the report and it was as if I was looking across the table. She was introverted, sensitive, caring, judgmental and liked rules. According to the tests no two people in all of creation were more opposite. She was introverted, I like a party. She was sensitive and caring and I liked to argue. I am objective and rational, she follows her feelings. She likes rules and I say "what rules". She likes guidelines and deadlines and I lean toward keeping my options open.

I argued that this new found information may create further controversy in our lives and we best ignore it and move on with our lives. However near the end of the report it offered insight into which personalities may actually be the most compatible in real life. Despite our opposite approaches to decision making we complimented each other perfectly. The weak areas of one were bolstered and reinforced by the strengths of the other.

Now if she will just throw out the rules and stop judging me, I will promise to stop arguing and work on the details. There just might be a chance we could live happily ever after. Maybe there is something to this online dating stuff.

Politically Incorrect

November 22, 2013 commemorated the 50th anniversary of the tragic assassination of JFK. 11/22/1963 was a day that forever changed America and the way Americans view their elected officials. Despite an exhaustive investigation into the events surrounding the shooting of President Kennedy, the Warren Commission was criticized and questioned to the extent that numerous conspiracy theories remain to this day. Prior to this, politics was generally respected and there was a civility in the ranks. Despite differences that have always existed, opposing political parties were able to work through issues without causing a government shutdown.

The 1960's and 1970's were a tumultuous time. It was a time when many questioned authority and many reacted in violent protests against authority. College campuses became little war zones reacting to news from Vietnam and Cambodia. Individuals such as Timothy Leary encouraged us to "Tune in, turn on and drop out" and "Think for yourself and question authority".

It is from those times we have arrived into our present state of affairs. While I don't consider myself politically motivated, I certainly harbor my own opinions, I have had the privilege of meeting many who have had strong and differing opinions. In some cases these opinions have resulted on interesting conditions

Larry (not his real name) came to me with a rash. He itched and scratched until he could stand it no more. We tried lotions, creams, pills, diet changes and new clothes and nothing seemed to work for more than a brief time. Referrals to dermatologists and allergy testing likewise revealed no lasting results. Finally, in desperation we considered emotional issues. It was there that we finally began to make headway. It was during the time of the first Gulf War and Larry was frustrated and angry about the entire situation. He noticed that whenever the subject of the war arose his rash would worsen. He became intensely pruritic whenever he listened to President Bush address the nation. Once we put the pieces together the diagnosis was simple.

Fast forward a few years and I had the unique opportunity of meeting his brother. Bob (also not his real name) presented with a rash. We discussed the usual areas of concern such as new clothes, new pets in the house, new soaps or lotions etc. and nothing became clear. I recommended a trial of allergy medications and if that didn't work he would return at a later time for reevaluation.

He returned in a few weeks requesting further treatment as nothing was working. It was during that follow up visit I decided to bring up politics. "How is your brother?" "Fine, Why?" "Don't you work together?" "Yah, we work together most of the time, no problems."

"Do you ever discuss politics when you work together?" At that comment he paused in thought before continuing. "Larry and I get along great and can discuss nearly anything but politics. We have simply agreed to never-ever talk politics. Why do you ask?"

Things were beginning to make sense to me now but before I could label him with the diagnosis I needed some more information. "What do you think about President Obama?" He clenched his jaws and cracked his knuckles and I saw his finger nails blanche just a bit and he pressed them together. Before he could answer I leaned forward reassured him that I had the answer to his problems.

"Bob, don't laugh at what I am about to tell you but now it all makes sense. Larry is allergic to George Bush and you are allergic to Barrack Obama. Your rash will be over with the next election."

Priceless

Traveling has always been an interest of ours. Regardless of the time of year or destination we try to take it all in and enjoy what each location has to offer. I like to think that we are just as comfortable in a jostling float plane with foggy duct taped windows in a rain storm as we are during a five star dining experience aboard a sailing yacht in the sparkling Caribbean. I want to believe we enjoy strange sounding delicacies in strange countries as much as we relish a good north woods Friday night fish fry. I try to convince myself that the prices I am paying when I travel are really not much different than it would be at home so I shouldn't complain and just enjoy my time away.

Time differences remain one of the most difficult obstacles to overcome. A driving trip usually helps to offset the time zone differences due to the relatively slow rate of change. It takes 24 hours to drive from here to Denver and in that time you have only jumped one time zone. Contrast this with airline travel. In that same 24 hour time frame you can hop aboard a 747 and find yourself on the opposite side of the world a full 12 hours different in time. Despite traveling for 24 hours you will discover that you have actually lost an additional day due to crossing the international dateline. However, it becomes somewhat hard to believe when you return. You will regain the day and possibly even arrive home before you left! If you don't believe me, try it some time.

Paying for the trip becomes another issue that is hard to grasp. If everything were always priced in the same currency you could easily compare to determine if the price you are paying is reasonable. If you have traveled much you will soon discover that any price you are asked to pay is usually not reasonable, in fact it is often outrageous. If your travel plans have taken you to more places than Minnesota you will find widely varying prices that have no basis in reality. In Thailand for example, we could feed an entire group of people endless amounts of food and drink for a total amount of less than $20. Compare that to the chic island of St. Barthelemy in the Caribbean. As one of the French West Indies it has a reputation for attracting the rich and famous. Some of the big name stars like to spend their time and money on the island staying in locations that charge up to $25,000 per night. We limited our expenditures on the island and just enjoyed lunch in an open air restaurant. It was the best $45 dollar hamburger I have ever eaten, however I have had many $6 hamburgers that were much better.

Comparing prices is always interesting when you look at essentials and not luxury items such as hamburgers touched by a French chef. Last year when we were in Copenhagen, Denmark, I did some quick calculating on the price of gasoline. Correcting liters into gallons and Danish Kroners into dollars, it was clear they were paying a much steeper price, somewhere around $11.50 per gallon most of that in the form of taxes. Apparently, they enjoy paying astronomical prices for everything because the government will take care of everyone from cradle to grave. I decided that being unemployed in Denmark is not such a bad thing but having a job in Denmark could be quite an expensive undertaking. I guess it all depends on your perspective.

I really do enjoy experiencing other people, cultures and countries and I am not in the habit of complaining about the prices because it is dependent on numerous variables. But when it is all said and done there is something that is worth every penny and I long for at the end of every trip. Michael Buble' is a popular singer who has recorded a song entitled "Home". In it he captures the true longing of the traveler. "Another winter day has come and gone away in either Paris or Rome, and I want to go home, Let me go home"

To paraphrase a popular advertisement for a credit card, "A hamburger in St. Barth's-$45; Airline tickets to get there-$1500; Sleeping in my own bed, in my own home-priceless". Dorothy really was right, there is no place like home.

Pursuing Ordinary

I have been to the mountain top. Perched with friends on the edge of an extinct volcano crater we greeted the first feeble rays of sunlight breaking over the horizon of the Pacific. Snorkeling in those same aqua waters I witnessed massive sea turtles rising out of the coral reefs like alien space ships and silently drift into the azure depths. Dolphins by the hundreds broke the surface around our boat with exuberance, displaying sheer delight in their race through the sea foam. I have witnessed ducks and geese by the thousands gathering for their annual migrations. I have stared into the gaping mouth of a large black bear at a distance of 3 feet wondering which limb I must sacrifice if I want to live another day. I have seen the unusual and experienced the once in a lifetime events. I have known fear, excitement and exhilaration. I have traveled to many corners of the world and I have the desire to see many more. I have seen the exceptional and lived the extraordinary but in the end of it all I realized it is the ordinary I have been searching for all along.

Somehow along the way I have become somewhat jaded and cynical with life around me. I care, I really do. I am very investing in my family and friends and am desperately concerned for their wellbeing. I am concerned about my community and even the world at large. However, for every person who accepts you as you are there appears a line of people working on ways to influence, manipulate or change you to suit their needs not yours. What ever happened to contentment? When are we satisfied?

I recently attended a leadership conference. It is the type of conference designed to make you feel uncomfortable with your current situation and stimulate you to make decisions leading out of the mundane and into their definition of significance. I left wondering "If perfection is unattainable when have we achieved enough? What is enough?"

Sometime in the past I entered into the nebulous dimension known as middle age. It is a bit older than a young adult but a bit younger than a retired person. It is defined by an uneasy situation of still caring for your own children and launching them into the world, worrying about your aging parents and their needs and looking anxiously at your own situation. With one cautiously fixed on a dwindling retirement account and the other eye fixed on a crumbling world situation it leaves you wondering about many things.

This morning at breakfast I asked my wife if she was content. Not a simple "how's your coffee" type of satisfaction but a real deep sense of how do you view your life. Without hesitation she reaffirmed her sense of contentment. I am usually the first to reach the kitchen in the morning, not because I have a stronger desire for coffee but I have short hair and there is no need to style it. While she was getting herself ready for the day I poured myself a cup of black coffee and stared across the lake as the sun rose out of the east. I made toast. It was nothing special, just ordinary toast with peanut butter. As I sipped my morning coffee I pulled out a copy of Organic Gardening and Farming from August 1973 and glanced over the contents page. Planting potatoes was simple then. You didn't need a smart phone with a GPS to precisely design a garden plot. You simply dug a hole and buried the spud. I liked that. I like my work also but I wondered about the future, about retirement. Most retirement planners think you need ponderous amounts of cash in your bank account because you are going to spend your final years driving late model red Mercedes cars and searching for unique mountain top experiences before it is too late.

So many of us work like slaves in order to spend our later years in some reduced state of frenzy. We look forward to a time of less work and more leisure, less commitment and more contentment, less hurry and no worry. We long for a pair of slippers and a comfortable chair at the end of the day. We hope for a good book by the fire or a cold drink in the shade. More than anything we want a simple hug from a child and friend who accepts us unconditionally. After a long and trying week most people would rather relax with friends or go fishing or golfing or boating or simple mow the lawn and tend the garden. No one wants to go to meetings to plan events or programs designed to coerce others to do things they really don't want to do either.

It struck me that what we really want is to live ordinary lives, simple and unfettered. All of the motivational speeches, leadership conferences, management books and personal fulfillment programs we attend are designed to help us do the exceptional. And when we have reached the pinnacle and realize how empty our lives have become we hope to return to an ordinary existence once again. It was Thoreau that said "Many men go fishing all of their lives without knowing that it is not fish they are after"

To watch a brilliant sunset, to hold a child's hand, to laugh deeply with friends, to comfort those who hurt, to really enjoy good food, to feel the morning breeze on your face, to sleep well after hard physical work, to love and be loved, to be forgiven, to be eat warm bread dripping with melted butter just from the oven, to hold a puppy, to drink ice water on a hot day and hot chocolate on a cold winter day, to plant flowers, to plant a tree under which you may never feel the shade, to dance with your daughter, to receive a passionate kiss, to be intoxicated with joy, these are the ordinary things we long for and realize how extraordinary life really is.

Redneck Guide to Essential Oils

There is a virtual explosion of interest in essential oils. Touted as the cure-all for everything from apoplexy to Zenker's diverticulum, these miniscule vials of natural plant oils are becoming more popular than wrinkle cream at a Woodstock reunion. A quick search of the internet turns up 101 uses for essential oils and a plethora of places willing to sell you the latest, the best and the rarest essential oils of all. Some of the most expensive essential oils will rival a week stay on a popular cruise line.

Sandlewood essential oil from India sells for nearly $500 per ounce but it barely cracks the top ten list. For all you Pot-head wannabes there is Cannabis essential oil derived from the flower of the cannabis plant. Topping out around $950 per ounce this is guaranteed to promote relaxation and relieve tension. I couldn't imagine feeling relaxed if I accidently spilled my thousand-dollar bottle of Cannabis oil. The most expensive is "Champaca Absolute Oil" priced at a mere $2300 per ounce. It is supposedly the best at relieving depression. I can visualize my unbridled euphoria after plunking down a couple grand for a smudge of grease in a bottle the size of a suppository. I suspect the relief of depression is in the seller and not the buyer.

I must offer my own disclaimer as I have not used nor do I intend to use any of these above stated essential oils. Essential oils like acupuncture, herbal tea, valium and a week in Tahiti all offer real and placebo benefits. If it works for you then it's real. However, I do have some experience with real life essential oils and I wanted to share that information with my readers.

Essential by definition means it is necessary for whatever task or purpose determined by the user. For example, if someone wanted to open a bottle but didn't have a bottle opener, then the bottle opener would be determined to be essential. The bottle could be opened by other means such as pliers or teeth (if the intended user has any) and this may prove to be adequate however less than optimal but the bottle opener would still be considered essential.

Use of essential oils depends on the circumstances of the user. Some oils may be used infrequently but others may be experienced on a regular basis. One of my favorite essential oils is used almost on a daily basis, often several times each day. It can be applied topically if you desire to whatever body part suits your fancy but it provides the most benefit if ingested. The good news is that this essential oil is available by the pound and at a price affordable to the most destitute among us. Butter is the most essential of all oils and is all natural. Don't fall for the chemically modified oils designed to look and act like butter, they just don't have the same level of quality.

Butter is great at treating depression. Numerous unofficial studies conducted by myself over a 50-year span have identified the healing effects of a pound of butter. A big pat of butter on toast or a scoop of melting butter perched in the center of a stack of steaming pancakes has a tendency to prevent depression if used first thing in the morning. Used in the evening, it is best applied to king crab legs and lobster tails by dipping into small vats of melted butter. Who doesn't realize the enhancement of a pat of butter to a steaming baked potato or on top of a grilled medium rare ribeye steak? How about puddles of golden butter filling up the tiny potholes on an English muffin? Butter is among the most essential of oils. In the delightful words of my granddaughter Ella, she has proudly proclaimed, "Life is a butter dream". I couldn't agree more.

While butter may top the list of everyday essential oils, lard may be a close second. Rendered from the fat of a pig this may seem unappealing at first. I have heard from those in the generation before me that lard sandwiches were a staple. While not usually consumed in it's pure state it is best used as ingredient in pie crust or used to deep fry Canadian walleyes or catfish dipped in cornmeal. How about fried potatoes and onions with a healthy dash of salt and Frank's hot sauce?

Most of us prefer the spicy version of lard known as bacon grease. Smoked with mesquite or hickory and doused with liberal quantities of salt and other unnamed preservatives to enhance the flavor and enjoyment it is certain be included in your list of most favored essential oils. Moderation is the key with lard and bacon grease. It is best not to be consumed on a daily basis but as an essential oil, if used properly it can enhance your quality of life.

The best non-edible essential oil is an old standby in garages across mechanical world. WD-40 in its classic blue aerosol can essential at several levels. As a lubricant it is easy to use to loosen up rusty tools, bolts and squeaky door hinges. There is a report from Asia where a bus driver used WD-40 to loosen a python snake that was tightly wound around some portion of the under carriage of his bus. I guess that would be called snake oil. Many anglers have learned that WD-40 can be used very successfully as a fish attractant. A couple of discreet squirts on your fishing lure and you are sure to claim bragging rights from your friends.

The most unusual use of WD-40 was reported by a friend of mine. He was a small engine mechanic and used liberal quantities of the lubricant in his shop. When troubled with aching knees he would simply spray his arthritic joints with a generous coating of WD-40 and rub it in. It may have helped to loosen his knees but it didn't do much for the rest of him. At his funeral he was quite stiff.

The whole essential oil phenomenon is something that has failed to grasp my full attention. I won't say it doesn't have merit. It may. I prefer to stick with my old tried and true oils that have never failed to meet my expectations. A pat of butter, a drizzle of bacon grease and a squirt of WD-40 and I am ready to face the world.

Remote Control

On May 22, 2012, Mr. Eugene J. Polley passed away from natural causes. He was 96 years old. While most of us don't know Mr. Polley, we are all familiar with what he developed. As an engineer working for Zenith he invented the television remote control device which is a precursor to our current multifunctional remote-control devices. The family has announced that, following the football season, his ashes will be scattered between the couch cushions.

The original remote control was actually a small control device directly connected to the television by wires. While functional, it caused numerous problems as people were tripping over the wires. That particular remote control was actually named "Lazy-Bone". Mr. Polley took this concept and developed a control device that operated on flashes of light. Different triggers or buttons would transmit different flashes of light that would be picked up by photo cells located on corners of the TV. If you wanted to adjust the volume you simply pointed the control at the correct corner of the television and pulled the trigger on the gun shaped control. He named his version "Flash-Matic" based on the method of operation.

Remote controls today operate on infrared signals. You can play games with it by trying to adjust your television by bouncing the signal off of windows, mirrors or any reflective surface. It becomes more challenging if you try to bounce the signal off of two or more surfaces at the same time, much like a two-rail shot in billiards.

There may be future benefits of remote controls which are yet to be developed although we are now on the cusp of discovery and implementation. Currently you can use a smart phone to adjust your furnace, turn on or off lights and even program your DVR to record television programs, all from a distant location. You can also access your bank accounts and pay bills, transfer money and monitor retirement accounts or other investments. While not utilizing the same technology, it still remains a form of remote control. However, the real benefit will be realized when we can utilize a remote to control our children or spouse or coworkers. Who wouldn't love to hit the fast-forward button when the boss is rambling on through an intensely boring meeting or the mute button when your spouse reminds you for the 47th time of something about which you no longer want to be reminded.

How about your children? Too loud? Hit mute. Too rambunctious? Push the pause button or the slow-motion button. Husband coming home from work late again? Try the search button. Perhaps the ease at which we may control others would also cause us a fit of frustration as others would use the same measures upon us.

I have found a recent situation that is somewhat related to the above scenarios. My father recently acquired a set of hearing aids. Now with the latest technology he is able to enjoy the finest in television viewing without bothering his fellow viewers. Others in the room can adjust the television volume to their comfort level and he then adjusts his hearing aids to the volume that satisfies him. Technology to the rescue. Ironically, he adjusts the hearing aid volume control not with a tiny twist button but rather with a remote control. That's right, he picks up a small remote-control device not unlike the one used to adjust his television and points it at his head. A quick press on the correct button and he is satisfied.

Ironically my mother has found another use for the device. When she wants to talk about something that she would rather keep confidential, at least from dad, she secretly wields the remote control. A sly point and press the button and he has no idea what she said. Now that is a functional remote control.

Scrambled Eggs

I need to make this clear; my wife is the chicken farmer. I am only the hired hand. I was resistant to the idea of a flock of feathered freeloaders but over time I have found them to be acceptable and downright entertaining. When we adopted them, I had visions of grilled chicken wings and bubbling chicken stew. She had visions of omelets and brightly colored Easter eggs for the grandchildren and therein is the problem. Grandchildren and chickens go together well; in fact, the relationship is a bit too cozy at times.

You see, children give chickens names of endearment. In our miniature flock there is Nina, Brownie, Big Brownie and of course the one-eyed, hen pecked, lazy, middle-aged rooster named Popeye Henry. He doesn't have much to crow about so he only yawns in the mornings. I had other names in mind such as Pot-pie or Drumstick but these aren't working out so well.

When chicken farming is limited to feeding, watering and collecting the eggs it is fun and rewarding. However, over the last couple of weeks we have had a change of direction. One of the brown chickens got sick and we were called upon to make a diagnosis and treatment plan. I am not a chicken doctor and my wife though she is an RN, is not a chicken nurse but she researched and Googled until she arrived at the most likely diagnosis. She called me at work to announce her findings, "I think she has "Nasty Chicken Butt"! That was a shocker to me. I had seen something like it when our kids were in diapers and it wasn't pretty. "I need you to catch the chicken when you get home so I can give it a bath".

I have always believed the proper chicken bath is when a chicken is reduced to smaller pieces and is combined with vegetables and noodles. It wasn't her plan however. I wasn't going to touch a chicken with "nasty chicken butt" so a fishing net worked just fine. The chicken enjoyed her bubble bath and was later transferred to the chicken ICU in the garage. Sadly, she departed to that big stew pot in the sky and our first chicken statistic was over (if you don't count the one she accidently dispatched when a small shovel fell on a chicken at night).

Then this week after returning from a quick salmon fishing trip to Lake Michigan, I was greeted with the sad news that Big Brownie was now sick, but this old hen had something different and I needed to examine her. I guessed that being an old brown hen was risky at our house. "Do you know how to examine old hens?" She inquired. I didn't answer that. I held the chicken in various positions looking for injuries or abnormalities and surprisingly I discovered a swollen squishy crop. I didn't know if this was abnormal so I had to catch a healthy chicken and repeat the examination. It was clear there was a difference so I went to my computer and searched for information on this condition. Sure enough, there was a diagnosis of "Sour Crop" so we formulated a treatment plan and she was off to isolation.

I remember once when I ate something bad at a restaurant and I believe I had sour crop and nasty chicken butt all at the same time. It wasn't a pretty sight but I recovered. We gave Big Brownie the same treatment, bed rest, no food, just water. I would find the chicken nurse on her knees with a syringe of water, squirting it into the beak. She assigned me the duty of massaging the swollen chicken crop. I suggested hospice for the chicken but I was only the hired hand and was compelled to obey my orders.

Several days of intensive care passed with flickers of improvement. I was certain the hen had one foot in the chicken pot and fully expected her to jump in at any time. Then I received the message at work. "She is eating corn in the yard and pecking at the grass". Big Brownie the freeloader was back from the dead. She will probably never lay another egg and if she is smart, she will likely feign illness so she can get another massage and be spoon fed by the chicken nurse.

I guess chickens, just like people, can get sick and with some simple care we might pull through. Just don't expect me to massage your crop.

Sicker than a Dog

Modern medicine is obsessed with numbers. We desperately try to quantify a subjective complaint so we can determine the best way to judge and treat someone's symptoms. Pain is a classic example. If someone presents with a complaint of back pain or a headache we try not to rush into any diagnosis or treatment option but rather we tend to observe, question, poke and prod before offering a modicum of care. Part of that process is trying to determine how much pain you may actually be experiencing.

We pleasantly offer you the opportunity to look at a numbered scale with a smiley face on one end and a frowning face on the other end. While you are writhing in pain from a kidney stone lodged somewhere just north of your bladder we ask you to give a number for your pain. On a scale from 1-10 your answer may be 47 or 99 or something else off the chart. That's ok because physicians aren't trained to actually believe what is being said. We know that the scale only goes up to 10 so we subtract and divide your number up until we arrive at something we can actually write down in your records. Sometimes people say things like @#$%^&* which means "I'm having a bad day". That may be about a 9 or 10 on the pain scale.

Numbers can be intimidating to many people so using an emotional scale or something more subjective and less rigid may be more helpful. In a previous article I proposed a pain scale that went from "Pretty good...Not Bad...Miserable...Terrible...@#$%^&". This is something we can understand just a bit better because that is the way we actually experience things. But how about when you are sick; how can we best explain your relative health after an examination? Animal comparisons might just be the ticket.

If you explain your level of fatigue as being "dog tired" I can understand that. I had a dog that was so tired he actually slept about 22 hours a day. He never really got over it and now he is sleeping 24 hours a day. What if you are sick, how can you describe that to your doctor? My favorite way to really explain is to describe your level of illness as "sicker than a dog". Now that is a mental picture we can all grasp. We have all had the unfortunate experience of witnessing a dog that has just returning from dining on sundried squirrel or rancid woodchuck. The gastric event is difficult to stomach. So when you describe your level of illness as "sicker than a dog" I get the picture.

Treatment options for this condition vary. Most of the time treatment is conservative, meaning simple dietary restrictions, clear liquids and if necessary then appropriate medications. If you are sicker than a little dog, these options are usually sufficient but if you are sicker than a big dog we have to be more aggressive. At this level we often consider IV fluids, sometimes IV medications and in the most serious situations we may recommend hospitalization.

Hospitalization is never an easy decision because there are many factors to consider. Insurance companies nearly always have a say in the process and they may debate whether or not you are sicker than a dog. It helps to justify your admission if you are dog tired and sicker than a dog although they will often argue with our decision process. In my experience most decision makers in an insurance company are stubborn as a mule. If they do approve your admission to the hospital they would want you discharged as soon as you are showing signs of improvement. However this may be at odds with your doctor's ideas.

If you go to the doctor's office when you are sicker than a dog there is a good chance that with reasonable care and a bit of time you may soon be as healthy as a horse.

Sleepless in Oslo

It wasn't until jet aircraft were invented, that we discovered jet lag. Now we can literally travel so fast that our bodies leave our brains behind. Before airline travel we were just tired. Now we have jet lag. It sounds more sophisticated and exotic if we have jet lag. It implies that we have been somewhere. I have a good friend that must suffer from nearly permanent jet lag. Just when his brain catches up with his body, he is off again while his brains plods along, sometimes an ocean or two behind. Such was the problem we recently experienced on a trip to Scandinavia.

Oslo Norway was our destination. We left Minneapolis in the evening with the plans to switch planes in Iceland. This was helpful because while we were delayed in beautiful exotic Iceland, our brains had made it about as far as Cleveland or perhaps Pittsburg. If we hadn't had a delay in Iceland our brains would have only made it as far as Detroit so this was helpful. After three hours of pacing the halls, looking out the windows on the treeless tundra and wondering if I really should try the whale jerky at the snack bar, we were finally on the second leg of the trip set to arrive in Oslo sometime in the early afternoon.

Iceland is an interesting country. According to a family tree outlined by my grandmother, I have a streak of Icelandic somewhere in my past. In Iceland, they don't have trees so I guess it was more like a family shrub but we do have roots. On the return trip we also had a delay in Iceland. It was so long that I fell in love with the country and bought a t-shirt that says "I Love Iceland". My wife has already threatened to use it as a cleaning rag.

Oslo Norway is a wonderful city full of Norwegians and a few others who fly in and out or come ashore through the Oslo fjords. The rugged, rocky shores covered with birch trees and pines are strikingly familiar to our own Lake Superior. In fact, when people speak, they all sound like they are from Duluth. We felt at home.

Our hotel was old. Apparently, they haven't built many new hotels since Norway declared independence from Sweden in 1905. Our hotel was wonderful in many ways except it didn't have any modern way of controlling the temperature in the room. One hotel employee explained that we could play with the thermostat all we wanted but it didn't change the temperature in the room. That was controlled downstairs. If we wanted it cooler, we had to open the windows. If we wanted it warmer we had to close the windows. Simple and effective.

Our bodies were in Oslo but our brains were still only slightly east of New York when it was bed time. We were exhausted and ready to sleep. The room was warm so I went to the 5th floor window and opened them up to breath in the fresh air from the harbor and look down into the street below. Young mothers, side by side, pushed sleeping infants in baby carriages on the cobblestone streets below. Several shoppers casually wandered into and out of the shops. McDonalds, the American dining experience was across the street and next to it was a dark storefront and a sign. Part of it read "Dr". I felt secure knowing there was a clinic nearby and we promptly parked our jet lagged bodies into the soft beds and pulled the plush down comforters up around our shoulders and fell immediately asleep.

Oslo is quiet in the evenings, but not at night. The sleepy streets and storefronts came alive after the sun sets. In Oslo, in summer the sunset is very late. People, laughing and talking crowded into the street. Throbbing music echoed in the canyons between the tall buildings, rushing upward until it found an open window, our window. It shook us awake and I staggered to the window to try and usher the noise back outside. I couldn't. The sounds of the street rose as laughter and talking erupted into yelling and fighting. Storefront doors opened and waves of powerful music gushed out, threatening to wash us away. All of this was happening in front of the Doctor's office below. I watched one man punch another and then slowly the crowds dispersed. By 4 am the music quit and I was able to open up the air conditioner again. Peace at last as I again drifted off into an exhausted sleep.

Do you know what it is like when you are awakened from the deepest sleep, when you are perhaps just a notch or two from death? Within an hour from the end of the last street fight, that is where I found myself. So deep was my sleep that I couldn't orient myself when I heard the next rush of noise. Jumping to the air conditioner, I looked down at the street below as a street sweeper made his way slowly up the narrow cobblestone pavement. It was then I noticed the true sign on the clinic below. "Dr. Jekyll's Pub".

Starting Over

Flipping the calendar from December to January gives us all the psychological edge, the illusion of starting over. We could do the same in the middle August if we truly desired but there is something about a new month and a new year that triggers a sense of renewal, of starting over. We harbor the thought that this time it is different. Gone is the old, we put on the new and resolve to change ourselves and a small corner of the world and make everything just a bit better.

The top New Year's resolutions are remarkably similar each year meaning that whatever we resolved to accomplish during this past year wasn't completed or needs to be redone. The top items are nearly always the same; lose weight, get out of debt, save money, more quality time with family and friends, more healthy food choices, and exercise more. Last year I resolved to stop procrastinating but I never got around to it. I also resolved to exercise more, unfortunately most of my exertion was primarily jumping to conclusions and beating around the bush. This year it is going to be different.

Statistically speaking about 45% of Americans usually make resolutions but only about 75% of the 45% keep those resolutions through the first week of January and less than half will make it through 6 months. On the opposite end, 38% of Americans report never making resolutions so we can assume they reach their non-goals 100% of the time.

In order to simplify my outlook on the coming year I have altered my personal goals to be less defined and could be summed up in a simple phrase; more or less. Perhaps it is trick I have learned from my lawyer friends, never get yourself backed into a corner from which there is no escape. By defining my plans for the New Year as "more or less" I can say with confidence that I am always on task.

I hope to read more good books and less bad books however sometimes at the last page I finally realize it wasn't as good as I had hoped. More good food and drink and less of the bad is a safe aspiration but the definition of each is always up for debate. More listening and less jumping to conclusions is an admirable goal but difficult to be consistent. Now after listening, instead of jumping to a conclusion my mind just seems to saunter around, sometimes it wanders off completely. More dinners served on the good dishes and less on paper plates; more marshmallows around the campfire and less leftovers in the microwave. I plan to have more hammock time in the summer and less behind the desk time; more laughing with friends and less complaining over trivial issues. More enjoying the sunshine and less worrying about wrinkles when I am old (my dermatology acquaintances may disagree with me but I don't care).

More time living and enjoying today and less time worrying about tomorrow is something we all need to do. Faced with a never-ending stream of dire political predictions, financial shortfalls and real risks to our sense of wellbeing we need to be mindful of tomorrow. However, in the medical business I am acutely aware of how fragile life is and how often tomorrow never comes despite our best efforts to prepare for the unexpected. I have convinced myself I should prepare to live forever but actually live like there is no tomorrow.

Reducing stress is frequently one of the top resolutions reported by those of us who succumb to the inquiries of pollsters. Ironically the definition of stress is directly related to the rate of change in our daily lives. Therefore, the act of reducing stress is inherently stressful. Since I desire to reduce stress in my personal life I have resolved not to make any New Year's resolutions this year. I was also thinking about resolving to be more decisive but I am not certain that I will make that resolution this year either. I guess I will think about it.

War Games

I am proud to be an American and I am also proud to have served in the United States Army. I am clearly aware of the dedication and sacrifice of our men and women serving in our armed forces paying the high price for the freedom we all take for granted. When I took my oath of duty I was made aware that I could be called upon to make that ultimate sacrifice. I am thankful it wasn't my blood which was spilled on foreign soil although in a different time and a different circumstance it could have been. We need to realize our very lives have been bought with a price. War or the risk of war is never a pleasant thought and we make our best efforts to avoid the possibilities of conflict.

I enlisted in the U.S. Army at the bright age of 17 and began my basic training at Fort Leonard Wood, MO in the summer of 1976. In that time, hair was a natural body covering. We were all into the all-natural concept of living which meant all body hair all of the time. Neither men nor women shaved and the hair on your head was worn long and parted in the middle. My hair was dark brown, nearly black in stark contrast to the stiff bristly frosted appearance I now display. Upon arrival to my basic training destination we had the privilege of getting a free haircut. We had the option of getting a long cut or a short cut but there was no visible difference. My comb was no longer necessary. I could now wash my hair with a wash cloth. The real casualty in this was the top of my ears. In the absence of hair, they became burnt and blistered from the sun. It was many days before the pain subsided enough for me to rest my head on a pillow comfortably.

It was during those days I realized my true position. I was nothing more than scum for the first couple of weeks but as we worked and trained together we became as brothers in a larger family. We ate, slept, worked and trained together until we could crawl through barbed wire, under machinegun fire and hike thirty miles through the night and laugh about it later.

I had enlisted in the infantry which means your job description is not typically available in the civilian world unless you are employed in an off-label position in downtown Chicago. We trained to attack and defend and when we were done doing that we did it again and again.

Eventually assigned to the 4th Infantry Division in Colorado I was stationed in the foot hills of the Rocky Mountains, under the afternoon shadow of Pikes Peak. One winter we again found ourselves encamped in a vast area in the southern part of Fort Carson loosely referred to as "Down Range". It was an area of devastation and beauty all at the same time. Our tents were pitched and fortunately I was then part of Headquarters Company so I was able to have a cot in a larger tent with a small potbellied coal fired stove. Several neighboring tents were likewise equipped and from a distance we probably looked some refugee camp patched together.

We had been there for several weeks and during that time frame boredom begins to set in. There were the inevitable card games and other such entertainment for the soldier but that wasn't good enough. One of my friends decided he no longer like C-rations (that delightful military issue cuisine). It came in a small box and within the box were several small cans all colored in drab green but printing on the top and sides identified the contents. It varied from a small tin of peanut butter, a larger tin of turkey slices and gravy, possibly some beef stew or any number of other items. Sometimes you found peach slices or applesauce or even fruit cocktail which was generally hoarded and traded for something of greater value.

It in this setting my friend cracked and decided that rather than eat another tin of peanut butter he simply sneaked over to the neighbor's tent and dropped the unopened tin into the smoking stove pipe. You have to realize these coal stoves were simply two parts nested on top of one another. Nothing other than gravity held them together. The peanut butter tin dropped into the fire and rested in the hot coals for only a minute. Pressure built and soon there was a startling pop and the stove jumped as the can burst open.

We could hardly contain our enthusiasm as we considered other options. What we didn't fully realize is that the neighboring tent was at that moment planning retaliation. Typical of most wars, this was on the verge of escalating. We soon found a sizzling can of jelly in our stove which promptly burst from the heat.

Back and forth went the battle until night fall. By then the little cans had all been blasted and burnt. We came across a can of ham slices in gravy. This wasn't your little snack size; no it was for the hungry soldier. Tip-toeing across the compound I slipped it into the first glowing stovepipe and quickly retreated a safe distance. The pleasant little pop which had entertained us all day was slow in developing. We paused wondering what could have gone wrong. It was then the can exploded. There was enough force to send the different pieces of the coal fired stove in different directions. Black sooty smoke filled the air and hot glowing coals landed on sleeping bags and an equally hot Sargent exited his quarters with murderous intent.

Thankfully the culprit was never clearly identified. All coal fired stoves were ordered to be extinguished immediately and we slept in cold tents from then on. We had won the battle but we lost the war.

You Can't Win Them All

Every so often in our lives we are faced with a situation in which there seems no way to win. Now I understand that winning isn't everything but regardless of the situation I would like to come out smelling like a rose. If I could dare to quote the Bard of Avon, "This is the winter of our discontent". To put it bluntly, spring is skating on thin ice as the winter weather just seems to snowball. Every other day I declare with confidence that each cold snap is the last and we shall all be attending the imminent demise of old man winter.

Yet I know that hope springs eternal and we will yet see Frosty the snowman pushing up daisies. Now I am no spring chicken but I do have a spring in my step and I certainly don't want to lead anyone down the garden path but I would like this winter to kick the bucket. Each time we experienced some blue sky it was really just the calm before the storm.

Now I don't want to be just a fair weather friend but the truth is every cloud has a silver lining. With spring we want to get outside and get our hands dirty. There is work to be done but we seem to be living under a cloud. We want to work but we are only able to sit around and shoot the breeze. We would like to say we have it made in the shade but the truth is into each life some rain must fall.

To make matters worse, we also had our sewer freeze up this winter. I would like to say we came out smelling like a rose but I can't. What's done is done and it's all water over the dam. Now I am not my brother's keeper but I got myself into hot water when I suggested every man for himself. There is no sense making waves and crying over spilt milk. I tried to take the moral high ground and encouraged her to stop making a mountain out of a mole hill. Even though I am just an average Joe, my wife is a class act and she is hard as nails. In fact she was flush with ideas but I encouraged her to just let the dust settle as this too shall pass.

As each snowfall passed I was certain it was the last. I have discovered, with winter, the sky's the limit. The wintery blasts of January and February were really just the tip of the iceberg. As we progressed into March and finally April I realized we were actually swimming against the tide. As each weather record falls we have discovered we are now sailing in uncharted waters.

Meteorologists like to call the shots but I rather believe they play it by ear and when they actually do get a forecast correct they like to toot their own horn. Yet despite my deep distrust in their forecast, each and every hint of spring was music to my ears.

I honestly believe we all got the short end of the stick this year. Finally, after what I believed to be the last snowstorm of the season I sipped my coffee and looked out the window on the deep fresh snow in my yard. My birdfeeder was crushed and broken and leading up to it was a long line of big bear tracks. To make matters worse he left an enormous mound of fragrant fertilizer near my front door.

I smiled to myself. There was no sense getting mad as a hatter over something that simple. There are bigger fish to fry in this world. I realized some days you are the dog and some days you are the hydrant.

Yes Virginia, there is a Santa Claus

I receive mail of every sort, of every size and shape and package coloration and most of it finds a direct path to the recycling bin, the garbage or the shredder but every once in a while, something catches my eye and I pause for just a moment. Recently I got a notice from the IRS that I failed to file a form from 2012, you know, one of those unimportant forms that no one really cares about except some IRS agent trying to justify his or her job. No, I am not getting audited or going to jail and I don't owe any taxes but any letter from the IRS still gets my attention. The delinquent form got filed.

Then I noticed a letter from the DEA, Drug Enforcement Administration. That always gets my attention as well. The DEA and I are old friends and we like to keep in touch. This time they sent me a Christmas card in the form of a renewal of my certificate. I am always happy to receive holiday greetings without any strings attached.

I dug through the stack of junk mail, quickly sorting it into recycling junk and just plain old worthless junk mail. Catalogs, drug company advertisements, throw-away magazines promising a wealth of knowledge if I would only succumb to the temptations between the pages and a number of other items all made their way into the bin. Then I saw it peeking out from the mess on my desk top, a small Victorian era postcard with the smile of a young girl staring up at me.

In September 1897 an editorial appeared in *The Sun,* a New York newspaper that contained the now famous statement, "Yes Virginia, there is a Santa Claus". Virginia O'Hanlon, an 8-year-old girl took the time to compose a simple letter to the editor inquiring about the reality of Santa Claus. This simple letter became famous because of the editors reply and eventually the entire story was made into Emmy award winning movie.

I bring this up because the simple postcard came to me from an old friend named Virginia, someone to whom I have not spoken in many, many years. It seems that there has been little to smile about recently and one of my past stories rose to the occasion of offering her a brief respite from some of the difficult things we all must face. In her empty house she laughed. Not just a giggle or a smile but a real laugh that replaced tears of sadness with tears of joy and for a moment made her feel good again.

It had been a difficult day up to that point. Overwhelmed by the onslaught of disease I was struggling to keep up with my schedule. Too often I felt disconnected from those I was trained to help. Sometimes you do things that are not appreciated, you say things that are misunderstood, you try things that may not make any difference and you wonder out loud if you really make a difference at all in the troubled world in which we live. Then you get a small hand written Victorian postcard without a return address and everything is better.

I realized for a moment that perhaps it is the small things we do in life that are really the big things after all. A smile, a touch, a kind word, a story without any purpose other than to make someone's day just a bit brighter, these are the things that really matter.

Virginia, if I touched your heart with a simple story, you touched me back with some of the kindest words I would ever hope to hear; that I made a difference in someone's life. "Yes Virginia, there is a Santa Claus".

Time for Breakfast

No other meal other than dinner or lunch inspires me as much as breakfast. In my opinion a good breakfast is a great start to any day. It doesn't have to be a Paul Bunyan sized breakfast to be good, in fact many great breakfast meals are wonderfully healthy and they don't have to be heavy or laden with grease.

I am the breakfast chef at our house. On work days I prepare the coffee maker the evening before so each morning we awaken to the smell fresh ground, fresh brewed coffee just about the time our alarms signal the start of a new day. Swedish pancakes, those thin slices of heaven laden with eggs and dripping in butter are my standard fare on weekends but lately I have been experimenting with an oven baked pancake when no two pancakes ever come out of the oven the same. Topped with fresh blueberries or strawberries and a dusting of powdered sugar it is fit for the Queen of England.

Going out for breakfast is always enjoyable. I have enjoyed many fine meals but the best I have ever experienced was in the city of Istanbul, Turkey. The tables of food filled an entire room. Stacks of different kinds of bread, local meats, cheeses, olives, dates, nuts, yogurts, fruits, vegetables of every kind were stacked in heaps around the room. On one end of the bread table stood a large frame of honey comb dripping with fresh honey. Guests would take the large curved knife and carve off chunks of sticky honeycomb and let the golden liquid pour out onto their Turkish yogurt covered in dates and nuts. Strong black Turkish coffee, stiff enough to curl the hair of most Scandinavians topped off the meal.

One of the more interesting breakfast meals I have encountered was in Thailand where we lived with a local family for 2 weeks. While they offered to prepare and serve us with a typical western breakfast of bacon and eggs we declined, instead wishing to join in with the normal family style of meals. The first morning we were served enormous portions of squid fried rice. Not having eaten squid before I found the tentacles to be a bit on the chewy side but overall satisfying.

We still have contact with several people in Thailand and I recently received an email from Crandall Jensen (his pen name), a friend of mine. He currently lives in northern Thailand with his wife who is from the country. This is his recent experience.

Yesterday the rice fields around our house (three sides) began the flooding process getting ready to plant baby rice. The rice fields are full of crickets that do not survive underwater. So, they all decided to head for high ground. "Wow" they said, "look at that house sitting on high ground with its light on. I bet they left that light on for us!"

Each called to a neighbor who called to another neighbor and ten trillion of them started for our house. Under the doors and into the bedroom they came wanting to watch TV with me. Large ones and small ones alike, they all came in. I was not aware of my friendly company until I looked at the floor - the floor was black. Black and moving!

I grabbed a broom and out they went, but not for long. In they came this time ten folds over!

I went to find Nuch (Crandall's wife) and her mother to tell them we need to put a blanket under the door to stop them. Do you know where I found the ladies? ON THE FLOOR catching crickets! They were putting them in jars!

"Why are you doing that?" I asked. "Just sweep them out the door!

"NO!" They replied. "They are going to be fried for breakfast!"

This morning I skipped eating.

I guess that gives a new definition to fast food.

The Music Theater

There is a secret place I like to go to listen to music. My wife thinks I am fishing but actually the fishing is secondary. It is really the music that draws me. It is a deep river bend with a high bank curved like a giant bowl that is open on one side, an amphitheater. The stage is a small muddy bank where you can stand and all of the sounds of the river and forest seem to reflect off of the high banks surrounding the stage. It was to this stage that I went on a cool sunny morning in June.

To get there you have to drive down a narrow gravel road and slip your canoe into the river alongside a thick patch of cattails. From there it is a short paddle downstream and around the first bend to get to the theater. The music was already playing before I arrived. In fact, in the north woods the music never really stops, the musicians just work in shifts. The harrumphing and whirring of the night shift frogs were signing off when the first whistling and chirping of the morning shift began. Somewhere in there a couple of eagles squeaked and squawked, frightfully out of tune. The mosquitos hummed along in harmony and rose to a crescendo as I neared the river bank. The staccato of my slapping did little to change the melody. The price of admission to this concert was going to be blood.

The dark green ribbon of the river was the music staff and the thousands of bugs on the surface were 8th and 16th notes scurrying to find their positions in the musical score. As I floated down toward the first bend in the river I cast my fishing lure into cluster of water bugs and stirred up the notes. The musicians responded and the music was wonderful. As my canoe bumped into a log along the shore two ushers came out to investigate. A pair of otters slipping in and out of the water along the shore rose up and stared disapprovingly at the intruder who would dare to interrupt the performance. They said something to me which I didn't fully understand. It sounded as if you took a bark, a growl and a chuckle and mixed them all together and threw them at someone. I didn't speak otter but I understood that I was to keep quiet. As they slipped in and out of the shallows a deer came down to drink. The otters escorted me along, making sure I didn't get out of line.

Just as I arrived at the amphitheater there was a great rushing sound above me. Two bald eagles arrived for the concert as well. One of them perched in the balcony section just above me on the river. A large white pine tree, scarred by years of life along the river bank, this was obviously premium seating reserved for those with season tickets. They seemed to ignore those in the general admission seats. I didn't mind.

Another chorus erupted along the side of the theater. A mother wood duck with her downy brood were desperately trying to climb out of the river and up the steep sandy bank. Like a kindergarten class on a field trip, she whistled and flapped and splashed desperately trying to keep the little fuzz balls in line. It was then I noticed the two otters slipping along the shadows in her direction. The 8 or 9 ducklings would get a couple of feet out of the water and then roll all the way back down. Like a silent cheerleader on the stage, I urged them onward to safety. I was certain that if the otters didn't descend on this family then the eagles in the balcony would likely take advantage of the defenseless ones.

I cast my fishing lure into the deepest part of the river and as the lure retraced its path to my location a musky swirled out of the water and destroyed my peace and quiet. My line was cut so I retied and tried it again with the same results. Another musky or likely the same one and another cut line. I thought I had it tough but I realized it was a tougher life for a little wood duck. If the otters and the eagles didn't get you then the musky might.

The little ducks clustered together under an overhanging tree as the otters went on their way. Out of reach of the musky and out of sight from the eagles they were safe, at least for a little while. It was time to go.

I saw the swirl along the old mossy log as the big smallmouth bass revealed his home address. I cast and he responded. We danced together on the river, he and I never missing a step, keeping in time with the music. After we greeted one another up close he went back to his home by the big stump. Maybe someday I will say hi to him again when I come back to listen to the music.

The Finish Line

I said goodbye to a friend today. I said goodbye every day for two weeks but today she went home. She finished the race and crossed the finish line. I don't know how she started the race or how she managed the middle of the race but I do know in the end she finished well, with dignity and humor and her family standing by. She finished well.

Karen was someone who grew on you and if you spent much time with her you were certain to grow as well. She liked to prepare food and she made sure you were amply supplied. You had to have an iron will if you expected to escape her home without eating. I would stop by each morning early to visit her and attend to her comfort. She shared her concerns and wondered what would happen to her. Would she have pain? Would she know what was happening? She worried about some things but not without hope. She expressed the ideas of Woody Allen, "I'm not afraid of dying; I just don't want to be here when it happens." Her last dying wish toward me was trying to give me a pie. She was in her last hours and she wanted to make sure I was well fed and satisfied.

Cancer has a way of getting your attention. When your doctor mentions the "C" word you tend to forget everything else that is said. Your first thoughts are frightening. "I have cancer and I could die!" The second response is usually a rapid plan of action. "I'm going to fight it and win. We are going to beat this no matter what it takes." Sometimes reality hits us hard.

I have always said that cancer gives you something at the finish line that others don't experience. Cancer usually gives you time to say the things you have always wanted to say and write the notes and letters you should have written long ago. It often gives you a chance to hug your family and laugh and cry together. It gives you a chance to look at yourself in the mirror and stop lying to yourself. It gives you a chance to make your peace with God, your family and your neighbors. Cancer is tough to handle especially for the person facing the finish line but it is like a two-minute warning before the end of the game. It gives you a chance to reflect and prepare.

There is a sense that dying quickly and suddenly is a blessing, but not always. A sudden loss of a loved one can be very hard for those left behind. You never got that chance to say that one final "I love you." You don't get the chance to say "I'm sorry" for some stupid action you may have committed in the past. You don't get the chance to prepare yourself, to muster your courage and say what you have always wanted to say.

I have had plenty of exposure to death and dying more than I would care. Sometimes I think I should have been an ophthalmologist or a dermatologist. No one dies from cataracts or a bad rash. I don't regret my decisions and I have been honored to play a small role the grand drama of some people's lives. My participation in those dramas for some was brief and for others prolonged and in the end, I hope there was some sense of good in it all. There is often pain and sorrow and suffering but there can also be laughter.

I am reminded of a story that bears repeating. A man lay dying on his death bed. He lapsed in and out of sleep wondering when his last breath would happen. During a brief moment of lucididity, he awoke and was greeted with a fantastic smell. It was the smell of fresh, warm chocolate chip cookies, just out of the oven. He called out for help but no one appeared.

With great effort he struggled out of bed and crawled into the hallway and finally entered the kitchen. Approaching the corner cupboard, he reached upward trying to grasp one small cookie on the warming rack. His trembling hand outstretched and hovered over the soft warm cookie with steam still rising and soft melted chocolate chips on the top.

A sudden whack on the back of his hand from the spatula and his wife proclaimed. "Don't you dare, those are for the funeral."

Karen, you ran the race and finished well. You crossed the finish line in style. We'll miss you and to support your final wish I'll bring your pie to celebrate your life. Thanks.

The Great Debate

"**There** are two types of people in this world: those that like Neil Diamond and those that don't." This is according to Bob Wiley in the movie "What About Bob". I feel the same about political debates. There are some who like political debates and some who don't. I don't. My wife is more inclined to listen to political hopefuls than I am. I prefer a shot of Pepto-Bismol and a couple hours of stomach cramps.

It was somewhere during the second hour of petty political posturing that I had a flash of insight. I realized selecting a president has very little difference compared to the process of choosing a possible future son-in-law. It is important to note that I have had some experience in the selection process. I have three great sons-in-law. My voting record with presidents isn't nearly so good.

Consider this: Choosing a son in law is much like voting for a president because I always have an opinion but I am never quite sure that my vote actually counts. I think many people harbor the same concerns. One vote in a massive pool of voters seems to lose significance. Or how about the Electoral College? Presidents are selected by 5 or 6 states and the rest of us really don't matter. Picking out a son-in-law isn't much different. I like to think have some influence on the outcome but I am kidding myself. Mom and dad have a vote but in the relationship Electoral College the daughter has one vote that trumps everyone else.

The primaries are much the same as the early stages of developing relationships. The front runner of one week may be shuffled to the sidelines and replaced by the next front runner. As each candidate took their turns trying to make it to prime time we listened with varying degrees of feigned interest wondering if he was the one. We considered the discussions between candidates and when they would leave my wife and I would vote. With only two votes we frequently cancelled each other. Sometimes when we agreed on a candidate he would suddenly withdraw from consideration and we were forced to forget his name and consider other options.

Another similarity had to do with fund raising. The young ladies who were campaigning for their candidates were successful at fund raising. Unfortunately, we were the campaign financiers although we were successful at enforcing a cap on donations. Unfortunately for us, none of the viable candidates were independently wealthy and were able to fund their own campaign.

I tend to lack enthusiasm during early political campaigning. Political candidates come and go and we seldom remember their names until they have appeared in more than one election process. The boyfriend parade is not much different. I seldom remember their names sometimes calling each young man by the name of someone who had appeared and disappeared months ago. At times I would call them by the name of one of my favored candidates however this was quickly denounced as tacky or inappropriate. I finally resolved this problem by ignoring all potential suitors until there was a ring. For presidential hopefuls, don't bother me with details until there is a nomination.

I really don't intend to trivialize the selection process of either future husbands of my daughters or the selection of our future president. Each is incredibly important on several levels but the process can be smooth or frustrating depending on the issues and the candidates. I am delighted with the outcome of the son-in-law selection process much better than I can say about some elections but either way I learned to live with the outcome. I may listen to the candidates but I am not going to get worked up and I likely won't expend much energy trying to remember their names until the finish line is in sight. Perhaps during the next political debate, you may find me relaxing in a quiet room listening to Neil Diamond.

The Mattresses

"Going to the mattresses" is a phrase from the movie "The Godfather" that is often repeated and frequently misunderstood. In Mafia parlance it is an idiom meaning going to war. When one family would wage war with another family they would establish safe houses where people could sleep. Such a place was typically an empty apartment or home with mattresses available for war mongering families to rest their weary souls. How they procured their mattresses I am certain, wasn't by consulting consumer reports or going to the mattress store to try out mattresses. I could imagine Vito Corleone preferring the pocket coiled inner spring silk damask queen with the multilayered memory foam pillow top. Most couples don't settle their differences by "going to the mattresses" but rather by "going to the mattress store".

We have never waged war over a sleeping arrangement but we have had a few discussions. It has been written that you should never go to bed mad so we stayed up for two weeks. Over all we have been reasonably accepting of the other person's preferences when it comes to mattresses but after 37 years of marriage we have now tried nearly every possible mattress design or arrangement possible. We just bought the last mattress I ever hope to buy, primarily because it cost nearly double the sales price of my first car, and it has memory foam. I need the memory foam, my wife doesn't. She remembers everything that happened in the bedroom for the past 37 years.

The first mattress we ever owned was a thin veneer of lumpy cotton resting over the uneven frame of a hide-a-bed couch. We couldn't afford a bed and a couch so we bought the couch on credit and paid $15 a month on 18% interest and should have it paid off any day now. It was so uncomfortable it made me envious of a homeless man stretched out on the sidewalk. At least he appeared to be sleeping later in the morning than I was. Our second mattress was an ancient metal framed bed with cables stretched between springs attached to the sides of the angle iron frame. It squeaked and squawked terribly and no matter where you started your evening you always ended up in the middle. Getting out of bed was always an uphill climb. The mattress was nothing more than thick cotton batting stained from the 2 previous generations that used it before it fell into our possession.

The 70's were a time of transition from traditional to whatever seemed to be different from tradition. As part of that era, waterbeds became incredibly popular. We bought the waterbed mattress which was nothing more than a huge bladder filled with water and we built the bed. That's right we went to the lumber yard and bought some lumber and built the bed and it worked. Perched in the bedroom on the second story of our aging farm house we finally had a state-of-the-art sleeping arrangement. We couldn't afford the more expensive waterbed mattresses with internal baffles to dampen the wave action. We had the simple and basic rubber bag on a plywood platform. If anyone dared to shift positions at night it would set off miniature tidal waves that threatened to expel the partner or cause persistent sea sickness. My wife got pregnant during the tidal wave sea sickness years and later in the pregnancy she was unable to get out of bed without assistance. That coupled with the floor cracking from the excess weight from the water filled mattress made the decision easy. Out with the bladder and onto something else.

The next was an inner spring mattress guaranteed to promote heavenly rest and marital bliss. It worked out fine but it must not have fulfilled our lofty expectations. We could never quite agree on the relative firmness or softness of our mattress so we went to the sleep number mattress. In concept this is great. Each side has a pump that inflates or deflates your side to your desired level of support. In reality it didn't work for us. Our numbers were so different it created a divide between us. One side was like a hammock and the other like plywood separated by a speed bump. If one person was seeking to snuggle with the other it didn't work. Once you crossed the barrier to the other side you couldn't get back. I'm not sure if we are just hard to please but that went into a guest room and we next bought a nationally recognized highly recommended memory foam mattress. Somewhere around middle age most people begin to be afflicted with disorders of one of the three B's; bunions, bladders or bad backs. I have one of the three and may be on the verge of one of the others. I loved the memory foam mattress. It responded to your body heat and would conform to your shape without problems. However, it didn't work for my wife because she is too light and has no body heat, none.

Recently our daughter got married and moved out taking one of the beds with her. We had to replace it so we went to our favorite furniture store to look at the options. After much discussion we finally decided to buy a new mattress for our own use and shift my favorite resting spot into the guest room. It is a comfortable, soft yet firm pillow top mattress with enough memory foam to last a lifetime. We finally agree about our sleeping arrangements. We are done buying mattresses.

The Christmas Letter

Since the advent of computers, we have experienced a change in the way Christmas greetings are exchanged. Traditional Christmas cards with a hand-written note are becoming less common and in their place, are appearing computer generated letters and photo montage's that rival professional standards. Glitzy photos that are cropped, rotated and retouched to remove blemishes and wrinkles make all appear as if we had cosmetic surgery during the past year. Almost anyone with basic computer skills and internet access can now plan, produce and publish cards and even professional appearing photo books at reasonable expense.

While the appearance of greeting cards has changed considerably the content of the traditional Christmas letter has remained about the same. As long as there are relatives, you will get to review in detail the medley of events beginning shortly after they mailed you the Christmas letter last year. These letters often follow two primary forms. If the writer has children still in school you will frequently get the proud parent perspective. "Our wonderful children are the best at everything they do. Sis has been doing advanced algebra story problems since she was 3 years old. She had to give up ballet lessons because she will be performing her 5th piano concerto at Carnegie Hall next month. We are negotiating with the school board to get her into the advanced kindergarten group next semester. Bronco is our athlete. He is six feet tall now and has size 21 shoes. He scored 10 touchdowns in his peewee football league. It helps that we held him back a few years in school so he would be more developed for sports. He says 4th grade gets easier every year." After reading those letters you wonder why your own children are turning out to be such clumsy imbeciles.

The second form of a Christmas letter often reads like an appointment schedule at Mayo clinic. Meant to bring you glad tidings and good cheer you actually feel like sending them a sympathy card when you finish. The most cheerful part is when you find out that Great Uncle Rupert finally got over a bad case of shingles.

Many of the Christmas letters we receive follow the same format, usually with a similar introduction. "Merry Christmas from the Curmudgeon's. Buster sends his greetings too, but he won't be out on parole until June. We bought a big turkey at the Piggly Wiggly so everyone can come over to our house for Christmas. Cousin Fred says he won't come 'because he broke his dentures and will have to put everything in the blender. We expect to have a good Christmas anyway."

Following the introduction most letters then revert to a diary or journal of sorts. Sometimes it is a month by month accounting of the past year but more often it becomes a documentary ranging from illness to mishap or injury followed by the surgical reports. "In January, Charlie got the big promotion at work but because he was suffering from gout he got laid off and lost his job. It was good timing because with my hemorrhoid surgery and broken hip, I needed help at home anyway. It is amazing how everything works out. With all the money we saved by not driving to work every day we decided to splurge on Valentine's Day. With the two for one coupon and the senior discount if you eat dinner before 4:30 we had a real nice meal. Charlie got sick afterwards but the food poisoning only lasted a couple of days.

"We spent March and April in physical therapy after Charlie hurt his back shoveling snow. It was good that he hurt his back because his heart is bad and he shouldn't shovel snow anyway. That man is so lucky. We spent the summer inside because I have skin cancer on my nose and shouldn't go outside anymore and he gets hives from bug bites. We heard it was a nice summer."

The obituaries are next, usually beginning with family members that have passed on, but it often includes friends and distant relatives as well. "If you were at Aunt Melba's funeral in August you might remember cousin Fester. When they were spreading Melba's ashes on the back forty, some if it blew in his eyes. He got a bad infection and nearly went blind. Anyway, he died last week. The doctor's thinks that the infection he got in France during the war came back. All this got us thinking, so we bought cemetery plots for each other for Christmas. I liked the spot on the hill by the big pine tree, but Charlie wants to be down in the valley. He snores so bad we have separate rooms now anyway, so what's the difference. "

No matter how depressing the content, the letters always end on an uplifting note. "Remember to celebrate the true meaning of the Christmas Season and if you are ever in the middle of North Dakota this winter stop by and see us. We would love to see you all again."

Merry Christmas and Happy New Year.

Voices

I have had the opportunity to visit with a number of people who have heard and seen things that others haven't. You can debate whether these voices or visions are real or not, but to those who have had the experience it is very real. I am not talking about a shooting star that streaked across the sky and you might have been the only one to witness the event. I am not talking about hearing a dog bark in the night or hearing a bear prowling around your house while your spouse snores away the hours in happy oblivion. I am talking about hearing voices in the other room when no one is there.

Dinner time at our house is a special time. It always has been. It is a time to sit and relax without noise, television, telephones and sports. Not that we don't enjoy these diversions, we do, but dinner is a time to retreat and regroup. It is a time to talk not only about the mundane and routine events of the day but also about thoughts and dreams and ideas. It is a time to celebrate food and family.

I know this sounds a bit like Christmas dinner every day but really it is a simple time to relax away from the pressures of life outside. The kids have grown into their own families and yet even when it is just my wife and I we treat our evening meal as a quiet time together. We might have a candle light dinner of leftovers but that really doesn't matter. Maybe the really surprising thing about this story is that a husband and wife can still have a meaningful conversation after 36 years together. It was during one of these quiet meals alone that we heard it. We heard the voice.

It must be clearly stated, there were no fermented beverages being served and there was no incense of any type burning in the house. It stopped me in mid-sentence and my wife nearly let out a miniature scream because of the suddenness of it all. No music was playing; no televisions were on, no cell phones chirping from voice and text messages, there was nothing at all. Suddenly there was a loud and distinct voice of our granddaughter saying, "Momma!" Now that may not seem unusual but she was in her own home 5 hours away. I made the assumption one of the kids were coming through the laundry room door but no one was there. We searched the rooms for talking dolls, checked computers, phones and found nothing. It wasn't a sort of "did you hear something?" It was a real and distinct voice that we recognized as one of our granddaughters. Finding nothing we laughed it off and decided to call our daughter and let her know what had happened.

Anna was a bit surprised and shocked because she explained how they were just looking at a short video on her phone and when Gracie saw her mother on the screen she yelled out "Momma!" Gracie was also playing with her evening snack, a banana, which also functions well as a make-believe phone. Anna couldn't determine if her phone transmitted anything and I checked our computer for any instant messages, Skype transmissions, or any phone connections and I found none. It wasn't like we heard an unintended phone call as if someone had inadvertently pushed a button on their phone and called someone on speed dial. It was simply a little girl's voice yelling "Momma".

Puzzled by this, we tried to consider the possibilities. I discussed this with a professional IT person who works on such equipment. He could not imagine how this could have occurred without any clear evidence of a connection and even if there was an inadvertent transmission there should have been more than a single word, likely we would have heard background noise as well.

So, what really happened? I want to believe somehow her phone transmitted the conversation to our computer in the next room and we only heard "Momma" even though that sounds somewhat unlikely. If that doesn't prove to be the case then it must have been the power of the banana phone; A direct hot line to Grandma and Grandpa's house. I am really glad my wife heard the voice as well, now I am not afraid to tell her about the voices in the attic and the little green guy living in the garage.

How to be Humble in 3 Easy Steps

If you think you are proud you probably are but if you think you are humble you likely aren't. We tend to dislike proud arrogant behavior and are drawn to someone who expresses or represents humility. But humility is hard to explain and even harder to live. I recently participated in an interesting discussion about being humble. I have discovered some easy steps to achieving and living a humble life and I am humbly passing this information on. Use it wisely.

Try golf. I am an avid outdoor sports enthusiast. My primary passions are hunting and fishing but any outdoor related sports attract me. The advantage of these types of activities is that you can easily blame your lack of success on the weather, the fish or the DNR. You could fish all day and never catch anything and still be seen as an expert. We blame the weather as being too hot, too cold, too windy or a full moon or some other factor well beyond your control. But if you take up golf you realize what a miserable game it really is. I love golf and I hate it all at the same time. Golfers love to be miserable. When the ball bounces off of houses, into ponds and stops under impenetrable bushes you can blame no one but yourself. When you get one incredible swing and strike the ball perfectly and it flies in the general direction you intended, be proud. With the very next swing of the club you are humbled as you revert to your old soul-searching behavior wondering why you ever became seduced by such a miserable game as golf. I once ran out of golf balls and became desperate. After losing my last ball in the pond I tied a rope to a ball retriever that looked somewhat like a basket and tied the other end of the rope to my wrist. With a simple toss of the basket into the pond I could pull it back out and soon I was surrounded by the virtual wealth of used and usable golf balls. Then the rope became detached from my wrist and with the next toss it sailed out of sight in the scummy golf course pond.

Later that night under cover of approaching darkness I sneaked back into the golf course to retrieve my lost property. Hoping to reach or find the rope I probed the shoreline of the pond. Finally, when nothing else worked I simple reverted to my innate adolescent behavior and stripped down to my birthday suit and plunged in. Warm on the surface but cold and slimy below, I swam down along the bottom and finally grasped the object of my efforts. The rope was firmly in my hand and I looked like the creature from the black lagoon as I crawled out through the algae and duck week and onto the bank. Since I had no intention of traversing the golf course in the buff I ran from tee to green swatting mosquitos until I was dry enough to get dressed. Golf is a humbling experience.

Get married. It has been written that love is blind but marriage is an eye opener. I couldn't agree more. My wife is my best friend and has been for more than 40 years. I help her to remain humble. She has much to be proud of and rightly so. She dresses well, she takes care of herself and she is well respected within the community. I used to think I put my pants on differently than everyone else. One evening as I undressed to go to bed, she burst into laughter. It is humbling to be the object of mirth when you are taking your clothes off. Between chortling and giggles she informed me I had been wearing my underwear inside out. I tried to explain how it fit better that way, she didn't believe me. I found out that I really do put my pants on different than everyone else.

Have kids. The people with the most wisdom and best advice about raising children are those who have never had a child. I am always amused by first time expectant parents. They huddle around parenting books and can recite entire chapters verbatim as if it were gospel. They plan the child's life of no sugar, no red dye, no processed foods and only organic unbleached cotton diapers woven by hand and air dried in the wafting breezes of the back yard. You can lovingly make the best meal possible but your toddler will reject it and choose the dog food every time. By the time the second or third child arrives it is store bought cookies and a Mountain Dew in front of another video so you can get the laundry done. Constipation is welcomed because you get a few more moments alone behind the locked bathroom door. You rip the pages out of your parenting books to soak up spilled milk and wipe off boogers smeared on your kitchen cabinets. First time parents have all the answers and experienced parents humbly acknowledge that they are left with only questions.

Humility is expensive and those who have it have likely paid full price. It never comes at a discount. But ironically, they never realize what they have because they are too busy helping someone else out of a mess.

Chapter 1-- *If There's a Will, by* John W. Ingalls, © 2017. Available now on Amazon.com or Kindle books.

Chapter 1

Hot Air

Not all those who wander are lost. —J. R. R. Tolkien

Roy and Lola Ambrose stepped onto the gangplank and never looked back. Roy reached out with both arms, gripping the handrails to keep from falling. After two weeks at sea, he staggered and weaved like a drunken sailor. Mentally he deleted 'transatlantic cruise' from his bucket-list. It was over. He took a deep breath and exhaled slowly, relieved to be back on firm ground. With the sea behind and the Canary Islands ahead, he lurched forward, anxious, and excited about the future.

The security computer beeped monotonously as his bar-coded ID tag slipped under the blinking red light. He blotted out the background noise of fellow travelers, trying to grasp the next step. He had insisted on a hot air balloon ride, claiming it would be an uplifting experience, but Lola wasn't so sure. He watched her smile as her ID tag flashed under the light. He knew she was ready for dry land.

"Do you have the tickets?" Roy asked. "I told you to get them, right?"

"I don't have them, you do... Don't you?" She paused on the floating staircase, descending from the ship's main deck to the concrete jetty. "Should we go back to the room and look?"

"No, we need to go. It won't matter anyway." Roy was feeling impatient. He reached forward, urging her onward. She hesitated, acting unsure.

It had been his plan, not hers, to cross the Atlantic by ship. They had experienced several sailing cruises in the past but always in relatively sheltered environs. Athens to Istanbul, Scotland and Ireland, the Scandinavian Peninsula. Roy's bucket list was nearly complete. But as each activity was checked off, he added others. An empty list held ominous implications.

Lola reached out and gripped a signpost. She must be having as much trouble getting her land legs back under her as he was. Tourists buzzed past on rented motorbikes. Taxi drivers honked and pointed toward them, clearly seeking riders. Roy raised his hand and waved them on.

Lola glanced over the garishly colored carts and kiosks dotting the stone plaza along Front Street near the harbor. The street vendors were stocked and ready for a fresh wave of tourists coming ashore. Hawkers aggressively reached out, grabbing customers by the arm and shoving wares into their faces. Lola hesitated as they approached the first produce stand. "Roy, let's get some bread and wine. Maybe some fresh fruit too. We'll probably need it, wherever we end up."

Roy scanned the options and stepped forward. "Nos gustaría...une botella de vino...rioja." He paused and pointed to his choices. His Spanish was poor but adequate for a tourist area. The young man raised his eyebrows and pointed to the same bread and cheese, confirming his selection. Roy nodded. His hand shook slightly as he handed over the money.

"Gracias, Senor y Senora."

Bypassing the big exhaust-belching busses, they walked directly toward a waiting van. A short black-haired man held a sign, *AMBROSE*.

Roy focused on their journey and felt moments of frustration over Lola who loved to linger and watch people. Along the harbor she had many chances to observe, too many. Hundreds, perhaps thousands, of Americans and Europeans wandered up and down Front Street skirting the harbor. Open-air cafes, wine bars and gelato stands called out as they strolled by. As she looked at the people surrounding them, some made eye contact, others looked away. One man lowered his newspaper just as they went by, and Lola caught her breath as she glanced at his short rusty red hair and dark sunglasses. The stranger returned to his reading. She furrowed her brow and turned toward Roy.

"What's wrong?" Roy sensed a deeper anxiety building in Lola.

"Nothing." She paused, looking back toward the café. "I...um...never mind."

Roy reached out and held her hand. Their eyes met. Lola blinked a tear away as she turned to follow Roy along Front Street.

"I thought you were going to get some fruit or something," Lola said. She glanced again toward the man in the café. A folded newspaper rested on the table, its pages fluttering in the coastal breeze. A bottle of sparkling mineral water, half gone, stood on the table. The chair was empty.

"I can't remember everything. You should have said something when we were there." Roy felt annoyed.

"You get so upset when I remind you. Let's just forget it." Lola resolutely looked ahead.

"Do you want to go back?" Roy fidgeted and glanced twice at his wristwatch.

"No, we need to go. They're waiting." Lola cleared her throat. "Come on"

The driver grinned as they stepped into the mini tour bus. "You ready for adventure?" With broken English and boundless energy, he jammed the vehicle into first gear and headed west on the dusty road leading up to the launch site. "Hang on!"

Hanging on was easy, but everything they grabbed, came loose. The rusted white van had a hole in the side. Dust, dirt, and exhaust entered and exited at will. Without seat belts, Lola and Roy clung to each other. They arrived at the balloon launch intact but dusty. The view was wonderful. The rugged hills and mountains stretched from sky to sea, dotted with red roofed, whitewashed buildings. They stepped hesitantly from the minibus as the idyllic mountainous landscape beckoned.

An immense towering orb of fabric expanded and fluttered above the roaring flames of the burner. The balloon waited, tethered like a dog lunging at the end of its leash, desperate to be free.

"Buenos días, amigos. My name is Juan Carlos. I'm your balloon pilot today." The stocky black-haired man greeted them with a wide toothy smile. After introductions, he went through the safety precautions which he described as "muy necesario," very important. However, the entire set of instructions lasted less than two minutes. "Any questions?" They shook their heads, no. "The main thing to remember is hang on and don't fall out. If we go down quickly, we will all die."

It sounded simple enough. Lola looked ahead, but she knew Roy's eyes were fixed on her. A tear streaked down her face. "Are you sure you want to do this?" he asked.

Lola paused and nodded and stepped into the gondola. Roy made it sound as if she had a choice. The time for debate had ended long ago. They were ready for lift off.

"Roy...No matter what happens, I love you." Lola sniffed and wiped her moist eyes on her shirtsleeve. He reached out and held her hand and said nothing.

"Roy, how can you always be so confident?" She looked around. "Don't you ever wonder or worry?" Roy swallowed slowly and said nothing. He squeezed her hand; she squeezed back.

The driver of the van and two assistants on the ground released the tethers. The burner, perched just beneath the opening of the balloon, roared, sending a massive influx of heat upward. The balloon responded. Silently they lifted above the hillside, catching a light wind from the hills, and drifted toward the sea.

They stared with wonder as the details on the ground shrank and the horizon expanded into endless blue. Far into the north, neighboring islands appeared as hazy hulks interrupting eternity. Lola slid her arm through Roy's. He embraced her. A string of brown pelicans and frigate birds, as large as kites, soared alongside, sharing the view. To their right the ocean stretched east, toward Africa. Yesterday lay behind them, and ahead was the great unknown.

#

The phone rang twice. "Bridge," Captain Caleb Beckett answered. "Beckett here." He listened intently to the caller and responded. "Have you checked their room? Is there a possibility they came aboard without checking in?"

"Yes, sir, we checked in their cabin and with security. Mr. and Mrs. Ambrose have not been seen or heard from since they went ashore this morning. All registered guests have returned except them." The ship's activity coordinator was concerned. The board of directors frowned upon lost customers, especially old people in foreign countries.

Beckett reviewed the scenario in his head. Missing or delayed passengers weren't unusual. Most of the time they were distracted, sometimes inebriated, but he had never lost anyone. "Check with authorities on shore to see if there have been any accidents reported involving an older couple with their description. We still have ninety minutes before we make final preparations for departure. We may have some leeway with the harbormaster but not much."

"We already did that as well, sir, but there's a problem. We checked with the tour company that handles our shore excursions. They told us, hot air balloon rides aren't offered on Tenerife due to unpredictable wind conditions. We also checked with their friends, the Nelsons in suite 205. They didn't know anything either. The tour company that handled Mr. and Mrs. Ambrose wasn't certified."

"Do we know who the tour operators are?" Captain Beckett asked.

"Local authorities know little about the tour operator, and no one answers the listed phone number. We are monitoring radio traffic for security reasons. An incoming flight at the airport notified air traffic control about a large brightly colored object, two miles out in the water. No flares or distress signals were reported. Search and rescue didn't find anyone at the site. They have been searching for several hours."

"Was it a hot air balloon?"

"Yes, I'm afraid it was."

"Let me know the minute you hear anything else. We need to file a missing person report. By the way...good job handling this. These things aren't easy." Beckett paused with a sense of dread. "I need to notify their emergency contact."

#

"Hello?" Luella yawned as she answered. She slurped quickly at her first cup of coffee. Luella was a night nurse at the local hospital. She had just sent her kids on the school bus and was trying to relax with a fresh brewed mug of Jamaican Blue Mountain coffee.

"This is Captain Caleb Beckett with Blue-Hair cruise line. Are you Luella Ambrose?" He paused before continuing, as if trying to gather his thoughts.

"Yes, I am Luella Ambrose, but my married name is Tinker, Luella Tinker."

"You are listed as the emergency contact person for Roy and Lola Ambrose, is that correct?"

Cruise ship captains didn't call to chat about the weather. Luella feared the worst. "Is something wrong? Did my dad have a heart attack or something? I told them to slow down...my gosh, they must be nearly eighty years old! Why are you calling me?"

"Ms. Tinker, your parents are missing. No one has heard from them for nearly eight hours."

"What do you mean, missing? They're old people; you shouldn't let them out of your sight!"

"Ms. Tinker, most of the time passengers get delayed or mixed up with directions, and eventually we find them unharmed. I'm sure we will find your parents soon. But I needed to let you know. We are doing everything we can to find them."

"Do you know what they were doing or where they were going?" Luella tried to think if they had left any kind of an itinerary with her. She couldn't recall anything specific.

"I am sorry to say, they may have been on a hot air balloon ride which landed in the ocean. No one has been recovered yet, but I assure you, we are diligently pursuing all options to find them."

A tight lump formed in Luella's throat. Her parents had done stupid things in the past, but this seemed more serious. She had to call her sisters. Luella prayed for the best but expected the worst.

Made in the USA
Lexington, KY
15 January 2018